I CAN'T REMEMBER

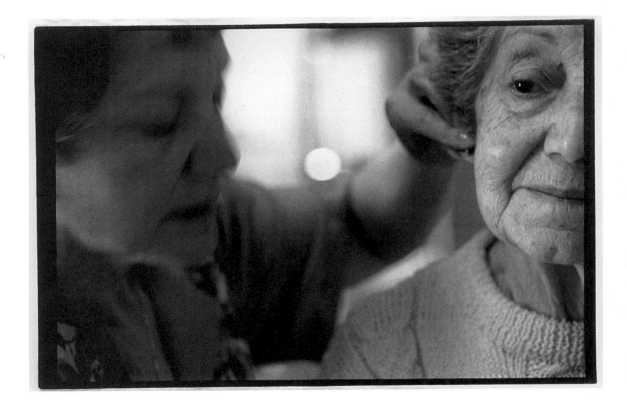

I CAN'T REMEMBER

Family Stories of Alzheimer's Disease

Esther Strauss Smoller

Foreword by Kathleen O'Brien,
Executive Director, Alzheimer's Association,
St. Louis Chapter

Temple University Press
Philadelphia

Temple University Press, Philadelphia 19122
Copyright © 1997 by Temple University.
All rights reserved
Published 1997
Printed in the United States of America

⊗ The paper used in this publication meets the requirements of American National Standard for Information Sciences—Permanence of Paper for Printed Library Materials, ANSI Z39.48-1984

Text design by Anne O'Donnell

Library of Congress Cataloging-in-Publication Data
Smoller, Esther Strauss, 1934–
    I can't remember : family stories of Alzheimer's disease / Esther Strauss Smoller; foreword by Kathleen O'Brien.
      p.   cm.
    Includes bibliographical references.
    ISBN 1-56639-555-0 (alk. paper)
    1. Alzheimer's disease—Patients—Family relationships. 2. Alzheimer's disease—Patients—Portraits.   I. Title. RC523.2.S63   1997
    362.1' 96831—dc21   97-1739

*To
my husband
and
his mother*

*Special thanks
to
David Hanlon
and
Marilyn Wechter*

CONTENTS

FOREWORD

To speak of Alzheimer's disease, one must talk about families. The disease affects every member of the family as they confront the physical, emotional, and financial demands of caregiving. Living with Alzheimer's means watching someone you love slowly become someone else . . . a person who does not recognize her children, or remember what he did an hour ago.

For the individual, the disease is frightening. Suddenly you do not remember where you are or where you were going. As the disease progresses, confusion and disorientation become the norm.

Living with Alzheimer's disease means facing challenges with courage. Once a diagnosis is made, decisions must be made about legal issues and future care. Feelings of denial, anger, and misunderstanding must be overcome.

But living with Alzheimer's disease also means taking time to treasure the good things that happen in life. There is always time to show compassion and love—to share and to remember before those memories are gone forever.

Alzheimer's disease is a progressive, degenerative disease that attacks the brain and impairs memory, thinking, and behavior. Alzheimer's plays no favorites: It affects men and women of all ages, races, socioeconomic backgrounds, and degrees of celebrity. The disease results in disorientation, gradual memory loss, personality changes, loss of language skills, impairment of judgment, and a decline in ability to perform routine tasks. The disease eventually leaves people incapable of caring for themselves.

Currently, there is no effective treatment or cure available to stop or reverse the course of Alzheimer's disease. The disease can continue from three to twenty years after symptoms first become apparent. More than four million Americans have Alzheimer's disease, making it the fourth-leading cause of death among adults. As the population lives longer, more people will have Alzheimer's. Unless a cure or treatment is found, it is estimated that more than 14 million people will have the disease by 2040.

The Alzheimer's Association was founded in 1981 to provide help and hope for families dealing with Alzheimer's disease. The association helps to enhance the quality of life through comprehensive educational programs, compassionate services, access to resources, and support for research. Knowledge provides strength for caregivers, and research holds the key to a future without Alzheimer's disease.

The pages that follow show the trials of living with Alzheimer's disease, along with the compassionate spirit and loving hero-ism of caregivers. Through the magic of her camera, Esther gives us im-ages that personalize the disease, capturing the daily challenges and shared moments that make each person and family unique. These pho-tos will live on—helping us to remember those who can no longer re-member for themselves.

Kathleen O'Brien
Executive Director
Alzheimer's Association, St. Louis Chapter

PREFACE

I was never close to my mother-in-law. Although she was warm and friendly and always bent over backwards to demonstrate how much she cared for me, I never quite believed her. At least not enough to feel completely comfortable. But we were comfortable enough with each other; neither of us wished to make waves. What for?

Since we lived eight hundred miles apart, our relationship was not agonized over. I saw her infrequently. She aged without my active support. But when she was diagnosed with Alzheimer's disease, my involvement in her life intensified. My husband was upset; he was confused about what should be done for her. I had been a social worker before becoming a photographer, and it fell to me to make more decisions for her than I would have anticipated, given our past relationship.

Her daughter, a psychologist, was too connected emotionally to her mother and was having trouble with objectivity. She was distraught, at times consumed with guilt that overshadowed her intense love for her mother. She, too, lived far away.

For months, we listened to telephone reports from my father-in-law, a man my mother-in-law constantly reminded us had made her unhappy throughout their marriage. In the early years, her three children had occupied all her time, and she had easily ignored him. Now that they were left with only each other, their arguments were daily and bitter. He convinced us all that she was demented and needed immediate attention. The appointment with the neurologist who would make the diagnosis of Alzheimer's was arranged in the midst of her deep depression.

On a Mother's Day weekend, my husband and I, my husband's sister, his brother, and his brother's daughter and her fiancé moved into my in-laws' four-bedroom, one-bath apartment in Brooklyn, New York, in order to evaluate my mother-in-law's condition.

At first we saw a very depressed old woman. She cried a lot and refused to get out of bed. "What's the use?" she said many times. When she was able to explain her depression, however, she made perfect sense. She did not sound demented. She said that her husband was cold and aloof. She could not talk to him; he gave her no support. She had no friends. She had nothing to do with her time. After a lifetime of caring for her children (she had also raised the granddaughter who was with us), she was left feeling useless. She loved to walk but at age eighty-four, she was afraid to walk outside alone.

She responded easily to our urging her to walk with us. She almost happily went shopping for new clothes and a pair of sneakers. She went out for dinner. She was practically her old self. It was as if we were witnessing a miracle. All my mother-in-law needed was some stimulation from people who cared enough to give it to her. Her dementia receded. Her condition had to be depression, not Alzheimer's. Wow! A happy ending to a Mother's Day weekend in Brooklyn. Depression can be cured! Or at least alleviated.

But, of course, that was not to be. There were more tests, more episodes of dementia. She was examined and re-examined. She did indeed have Alzheimer's disease. Her daughter, Arlene, now was able to take over the lead in making the decisions for her care.

Quite by accident at age fifty-eight, I had discovered that I could make reasonably interesting photographs of people. After thirty years as a clinical social worker, I had decided to leave my practice and concentrate on looking at people's outsides rather than their insides. I wanted to photograph some of the social issues that I had worked with all those years.

During that Mother's Day weekend I made the images that are presented in the first story. Then, later, following my need to present social issues on film, I asked the Alzheimer's Association of St. Louis to find some other families that would be interested in having their stories told. Hence the other two stories.

I chose the images for this book by the feelings that they evoke in me. They reflect what was going on at the time, but they are also symbolic of what happens every day in these families' lives.

In giving you these photographs, I am inviting you to share these very private, intense moments with us. The families who tell their stories here were very generous; they allowed me to take pictures of something not usually revealed in front of a camera.

I CAN'T REMEMBER

A Daughter's Dilemma

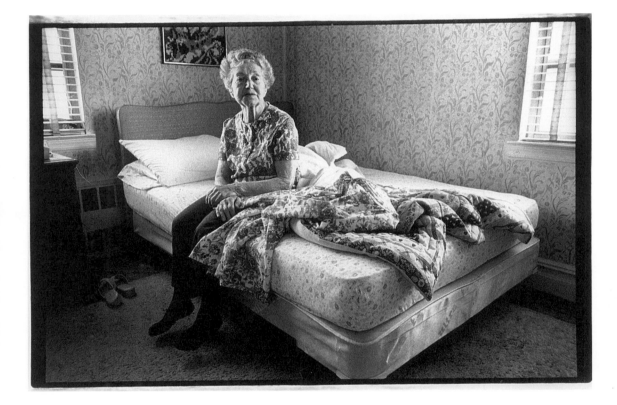

Lillian Smoller, at eighty-five, has Alzheimer's disease. She is able to let her family know what is happening to her, and it is terrifying. Her husband, Louis, and her son, Ted, live with her in a seven-room apartment in Brooklyn, New York. Her daughter, Arlene, tells her story.

Mom is eighty-six years old and is in the third stage of Alzheimer's disease. I first recognized a change in Mom about ten years ago when she became emotionally volatile. My dilemma is: How much responsibility do I have for Mom's care while maintaining my own family life?

I am a fifty-two-year-old married woman raising three teenage boys. My career is in clinical psychology, and I have a Ph.D. in gerontology. I seem to be the logical one to coordinate her care, since I am her only daughter and have the knowledge of Alzheimer's disease. But I left my parents' home in Brooklyn, New York, long ago and now live in Colorado. How do I manage Mom's care long distance?

Mom's role in life has always been that of the caretaker. As a young girl in Poland, she took care of her two younger brothers while her mother worked to support the family. Mom married at seventeen after immigrating to New York. Shortly after her marriage, she felt that she had made a mistake, because my father had a temper that frightened her. Never working outside the home, however, she was economically dependent on Dad.

Her focus in life was being a mother and great *balabosta* (Yiddish for number one homemaker). The standing joke was for me to wear sunglasses when walking into Mom's sparkling clean home. According to her family, she made the best stuffed cabbage, chicken soup, and coleslaw in Brooklyn.

I was the youngest of the three children, having two older brothers. My brother Marty was twelve, and Teddy was seven years old when I was born. My mother's first child was a girl, who died of polio. After my second brother was born, the doctor told her not to have any more children, since she had a heart murmur and had had a very difficult pregnancy and delivery. Later, however, she wanted to try for a girl. She continued to grieve for her first child and wanted to fill the loss.

I was the much-loved daughter. I modeled myself after Mom and loved her with all my heart. I was her confidant and listened to the hurt and sadness of her unfulfilled relationship with my dad. She told me to get an education and have my career established before marriage so that I would not repeat her mistakes. Her dreams were my dreams. Her hurts were my hurts. I sided with her about my dad until I was nineteen years old.

Then came the years of search for my identity in California. I chose to follow Mom's directions and finished my Ph.D. in psychology and then got married. I didn't fulfill the expectations of marrying a Jew and living close to my family of origin. Those years were difficult.

Then, nine years ago, I was shocked when Mom became

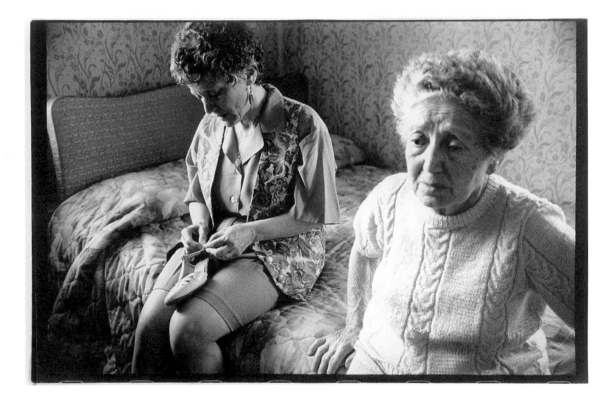

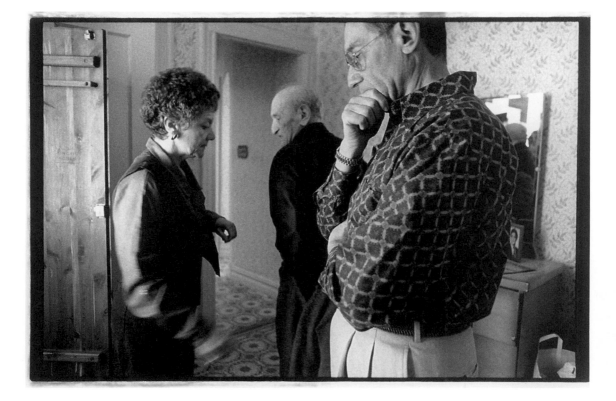

On a Mother's Day weekend, her elder son, Marty, and her daughter, Arlene, who live eight hundred miles away, moved into their parents' apartment to evaluate their mother's condition and help plan for her care.

paranoid if I talked to Dad. She said that we were saying bad things about her and that I was taking Dad's side. During one telephone conversation, I told her that I didn't want to come between them in their arguments and that I loved my dad as I loved her. She said that she would never forgive me or talk to me again. This was the first time in my life that she had ever rejected me. Even with all of her grief, she had always expressed her love to me.

The day after the fateful telephone conversation, she called to apologize and said that she didn't understand how she could have said that, adding, "That wasn't me."

Those outbursts became more frequent and were directed particularly at my father. She would say she hated him, he wasn't her husband, and that she wished he would die. They began to have more physical altercations. After a lifetime of frustration, her unfulfilled dreams were unleashed.

When Mom was eighty, we saw more signs of dementia. She and I had a standing Saturday morning telephone conversation. But she began losing track of day and time and forgot our calls. When we did have our conversations, I would listen as she struggled to find words to express her thoughts. She also began to cover up for her increasing inability to cook by saying, "I'm tired of cooking, I did it long enough.

Now people can cook for me." My father and my brother, who was living with my parents, recognized the decline in her short-term memory.

Mom always loved to walk great distances around Brooklyn. Now she would get lost in familiar areas. Her safe perimeters for walking by herself became smaller. She no longer went to shop. Mom became more depressed and stayed in bed longer.

Complex household-cleaning chores became impossible. The house was now dirty. I felt grief at the loss of my Yiddish mama, who was no longer the *balabosta*.

A couple of years later, her depression deepened. My father did not understand her, calling her *mishuga* or crazy. They had horrific verbal and physical battles.

In an effort to help, I suggested that Mom spend time in my home in Colorado. Before this visit I was in denial, convinced that she suffered from depression and not Alzheimer's disease. I had worked with geriatric patients who experienced severe memory loss with depression, and I knew that their memories improved once they worked through their grief and depression. I was hopeful.

I accompanied Mom on the plane trip to Colorado, and that trip brought me into the stark, cold reality that Mom had Alzheimer's. She did not know where she was or where she was going.

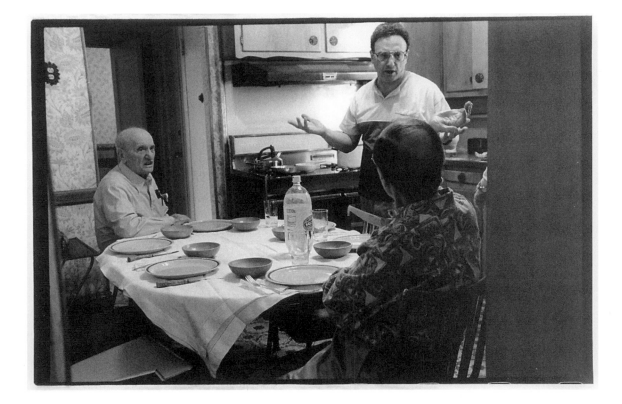

For months Arlene and Marty listened to frantic, distraught telephone reports from their father and brother, who saw her as demented, crazy, and needing immediate attention.

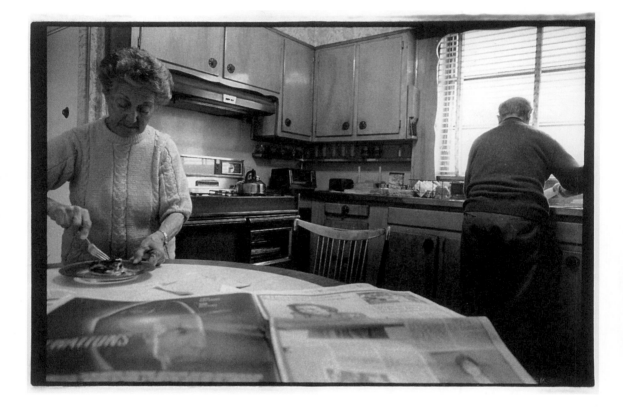

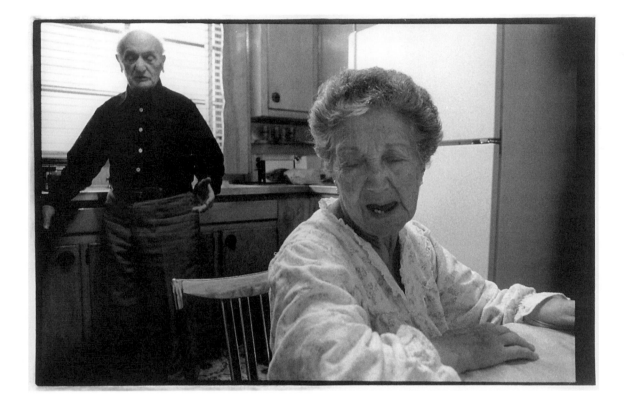

Louis and Lillian's marriage had (for the most part) been unhappy. Her three children had occupied her time in the early years, allowing her easily to ignore her husband. Now, left with each other, they argued daily and bitterly.

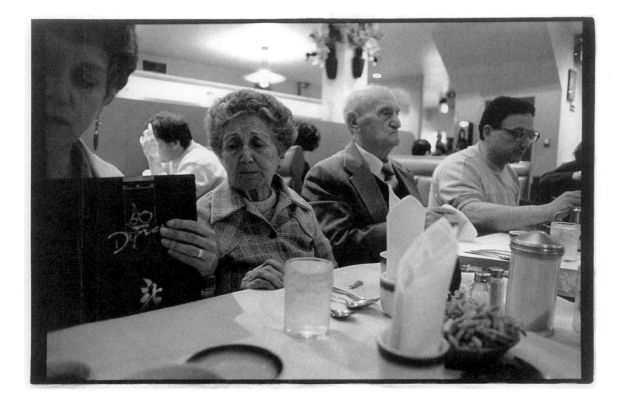

Upon arrival, she did not recognize my home, although she had visited me numerous times in the past.

She tried sleeping in the bathtub the first night. She said that she was trying to find her bed. She stayed for two months, and during that time she rarely found the bathroom, which was adjacent to her bedroom. We put pictures and a light in her room to help her get oriented. Yet most nights she woke up frightened. In the mornings, I found her in bed afraid and crying. She became anxious if I was out of her sight for more than a few minutes. One night, after a short nap, she awoke angry with me, saying that I had not called her to dinner. The truth was that she had eaten dinner two hours before her nap.

Gradually, because of my family's attention and my constant care, her depression lifted. My sons took Mom for drives and walks in the park, played the violin for her, hugged and complimented her. While I worked, she went to an Alzheimer's day-care program. She helped feed an elderly woman, whom the staff had been unable to coax to eat. Mom encouraged other patients to take daily walks.

Although she wasn't depressed, the symptoms of short-term memory loss, difficulty finding the appropriate words, and disorientation about place and time were still clearly present. Oh, how I wished

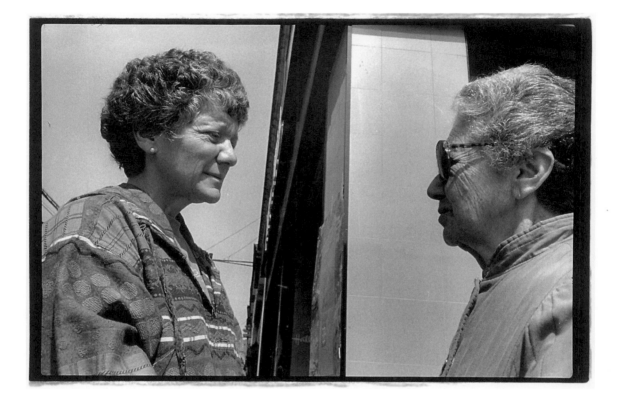

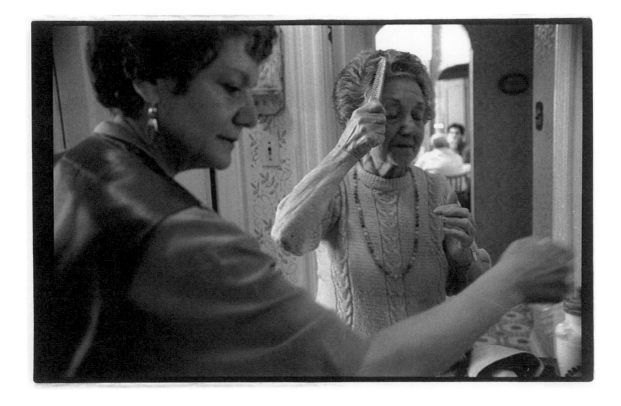

Arlene, who holds a Ph.D. in gerontology, can take a more informed role in deciding what would be best for her mother. But the pain is still there for her.

that I didn't know so much about Alzheimer's disease and could remain in denial.

During our first month together, I was feeling good about forgetting myself and serving her. I told her that I loved her and wanted to give her the care that she deserved. But I began to burn out during the second month. I stopped looking forward to the weekends when she was in my constant care. At work, I was helping other caretakers keep a balance in their lives, yet I found myself always putting Mom first. Many of my personal, marital, and family's needs went unmet.

Mom missed her home, asking more and more to return. So I took her back to New York. She recognized her home and could move around in it after resting. But Mom had great difficulty getting out of bed in the morning. She was overwhelmed by anything other than basic grooming and bodily functions. She was agitated, constantly hurt and angry with Dad. She became obsessed, relating that he never offered a kind word, was selfish, and had never loved her. "My mother told me not to marry him." Dad's reaction was to scream, "I can't take it anymore. I want to die."

Two days after we returned, Marty and his wife, Esther, came for a visit. That afternoon, we talked and walked; Mom appeared lucid

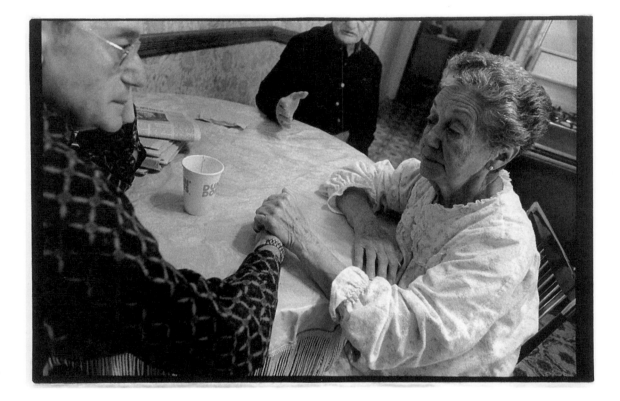

The family decides that a caretaker should be hired for four hours a day, seven days a week to help Lillian with getting up in the morning and eating regularly, and to listen to her upsets. An adult day-care will also be investigated. The caretaker will be expected to encourage Lillian to attend the day-care each day.

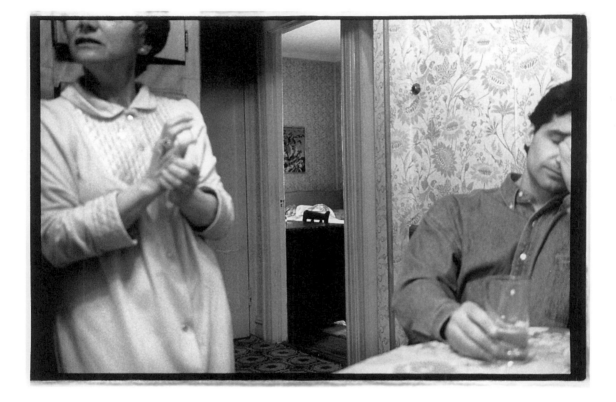

and happy. After dinner, which also included my brother Ted and his daughter, Sharon, whom Mom had raised, we talked at length, while Mom seemed to listen. As everyone was about to go to their rooms to sleep, Mom anxiously asked me to talk to her alone.

She said, "I don't know where I am. I don't know who anyone is. I know you take care of me, but I don't know who you are. I don't know who that man is who yelled at me. I feel myself in a dream. I want to scream and just get up and walk out—walk until I find out where I belong." I held back my tears and later cried alone.

Before returning to my home, I decided to write down all of the things that I knew would help others to deal with Mom. She kept reading the list of "To Do's," agreeing and telling me, "Only you can do these things. No one else here understands me." This response was a continuation of a lifelong pattern that we shared. I was her understanding, caring daughter who listened. I was always trying to make her feel better emotionally, but I never really succeeded. Quick fixes but always the pit of grief.

The next few months were horrendous. Mom was extremely depressed and refused to go to the day-care program that she had attended before visiting me. She was ashamed, realizing that her abilities and memory were deteriorating. Ted hired a home health aide to get

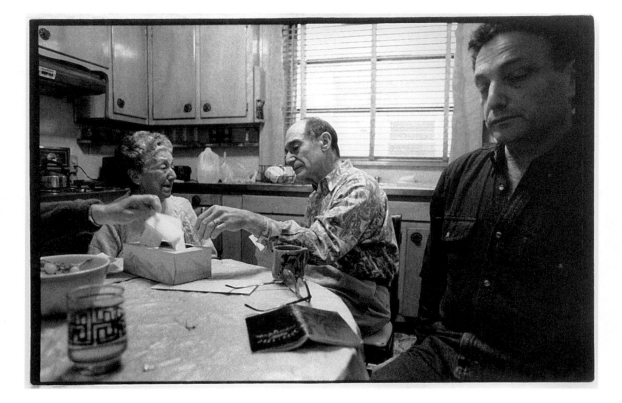

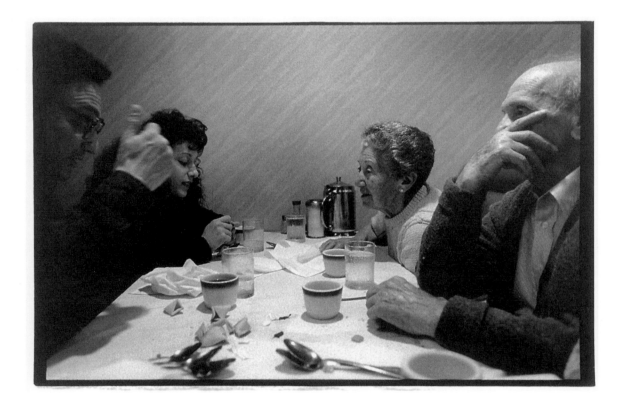

Ted and his father's strained and sometimes violent relationship has put a restraint on how much Ted can help his mother. Ted's daughter, Sharon, raised by Lillian, joins the family for dinner.

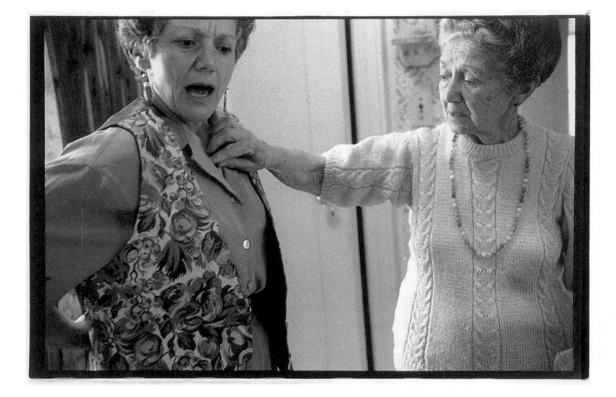

She is able to dress and groom herself and is still able
to criticize her daughter. That ability is always the last
to go. And her daughter can still react with age-old
anger.

Mom out of bed in the mornings. Believing that the aide liked Dad, Mom became paranoid and began to lock herself in her room.

I was two thousand miles away, feeling frustrated, and becoming ill from the strain and guilt. I decided to visit New York to get Mom more care. With much encouragement, Ted and I managed to get her back to the day-care center. In the meantime, my brother looked for another health aide. With the help of the Jewish Community Center, he found Louise, who proved to be a godsend.

I finally realized that mother's care was truly becoming a financial burden to our family. My brothers and I decided to apply for Medicaid to help Mom. Previously, her application was rejected because the title to the family home was in her name. This meant that she had a large asset and, therefore, did not qualify for aid. Now we decided to transfer the title to Ted or my father, so that Mom could get help. Dad resisted the idea, fearing possible legal consequences. But we moved along, with the aid of a social worker from Brooklyn Senior Services, who helped us fill out the forms correctly.

In the meantime, Mom's condition became more stable. Louise, the new home aide, had experience with Alzheimer's victims. Mom told us that Louise was like her mother. They hugged and kissed, walked and talked. Louise had a calming effect on Mom. What a relief

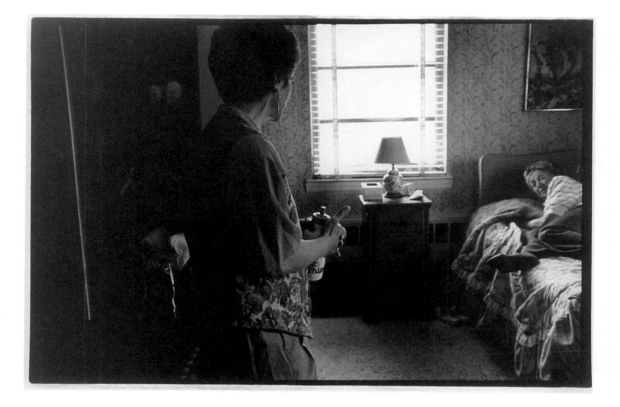

Each day begins much like the previous one. A reasonably enjoyable evening is followed by morning depression, anger, and upset. Her daughter cajoles her into getting out of bed. "What day is it?" Lillian asks. "I feel terrible. What's the use?" The morning is the most difficult part of the day.

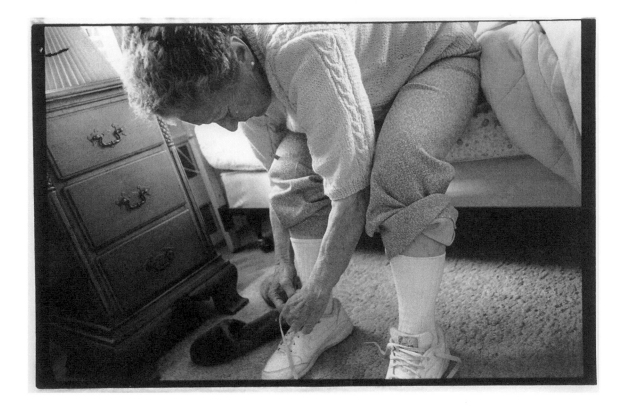

Feeling better as the day progresses, Lillian gets ready to join her family.

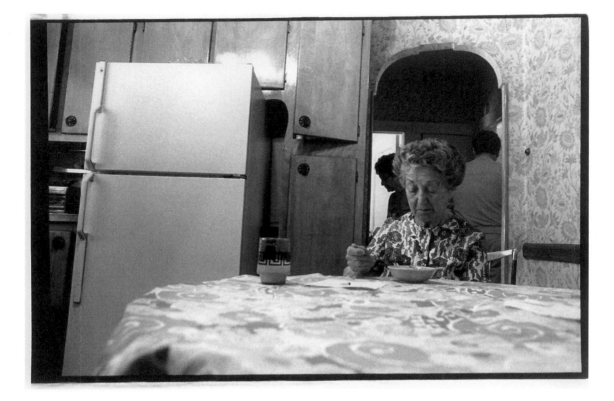

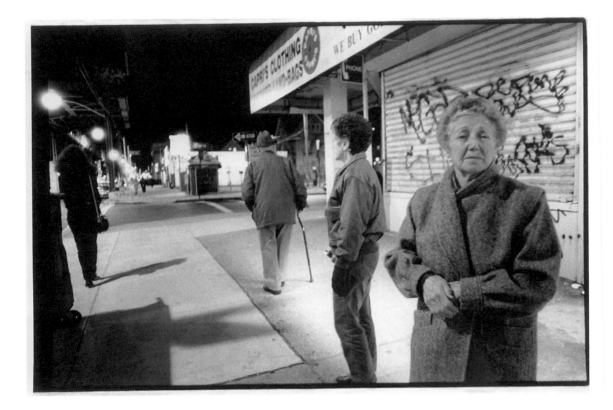

Loss, suffering, and lack of direction separate the members of this family.

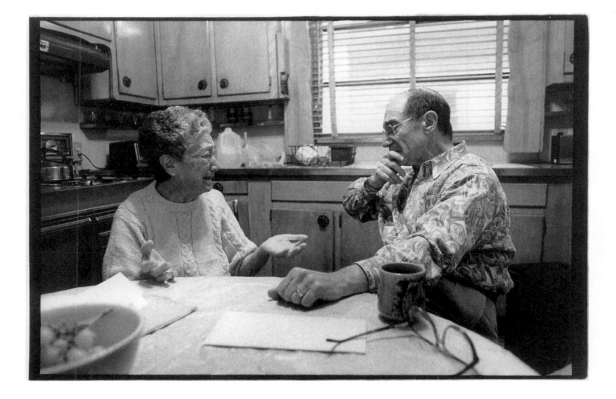

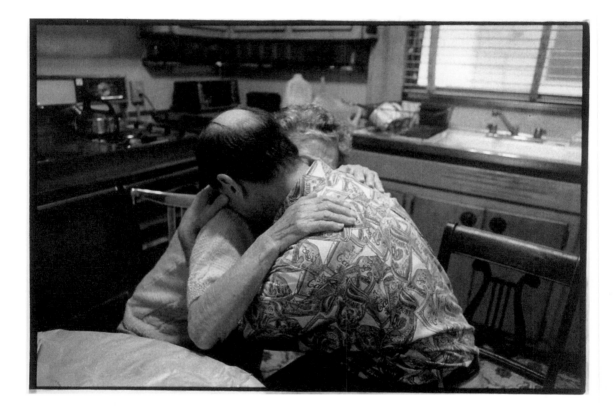

Marty listens to his mother describe her pain. An anguished Lillian tells her son that she knows what is happening to her. She can still think and reason and does not want to be treated as a child. "Please," she pleads, "don't call me crazy."

for me; I no longer felt that I was the "best" person to care for my mother.

Frustration began to return with my family's continued indecisiveness over the title to the house. Moreover, Ted and Dad were both experiencing physical problems, which meant that they would be unable to provide Mom with as much home care as she needed. After consulting with Mom's doctor, a lawyer, and the social worker, we agreed to transfer ownership of the house to Dad.

The Medicaid process began a third time. After an interview, the authorities said that a Medicaid card would be forthcoming. In the meantime, we are not sure of the number of home-care hours to be provided or whether Louise's credentials will meet the standards of the program. It is difficult for Alzheimer's patients to adjust to changes, so we are providing the agency with strong arguments to retain Louise.

I have noticed an improvement in Mother's memory for short-term events. But, sadly, she has recognized me less and less with each visit. She is painfully aware of her inability to recognize people. She says, "I don't want my mind to do these things. I know I have a daughter named Arlene, but I don't recognize who you are. I can just walk away and get lost and not know anything. I need someone to be with me all the time, and it will get worse." We cry together.

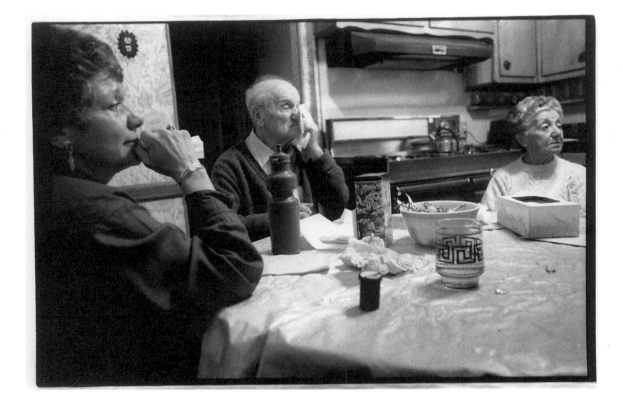

A very upset family listens to Lillian's pleas and her frightening and vivid descriptions of her illness. When she wanders away from the house she says that she is looking for her self. Who is she? And where does she belong? By wandering the streets, she hopes to find the answers.

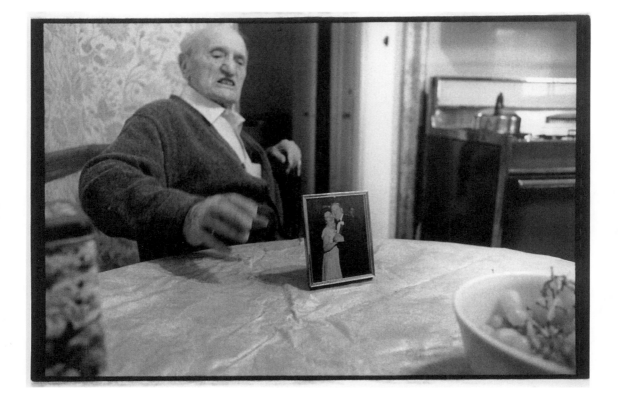

Husband and wife are caught in a terrible struggle
with an illness that shows no mercy. The husband is
confused and frightened, does not know what to do.
In the midst of his wife's tortured outpourings, Louis
brings out his twenty-fifth-anniversary picture and
tells everyone that next week he and Lillian will have
been married sixty-seven years.

Her caring is still strong. "I want to help others. If somehow through me people could learn about this illness . . . " I take notes of what she is saying, as she struggles to make herself understood.

Alzheimer's disease has profoundly affected my family. My mother was a woman who always liked to be in control. Now she seems determined to fight this illness and regain her control, but to no avail. My dad has had great difficulty adjusting to her forgetting what was just done or said. He is emotionally devastated each time she rages at him. He has cried more in the past five years than in all of his life before then. The illness has reopened wounds among all the family members. Old patterns, which I thought were long dead or unnecessary to resolve, are being replayed. At least we agree that our priorities are for Mom to have some quality of life and to be safe.

When is there some relief and peace? I find comfort when I walk with Mom and we thank God for the beauty in nature and her ability to walk, when she stops to talk and laugh with children on the street, when she takes pride in feeding a woman who refuses to eat, when she gently gives advice about how to deal with someone who is angry or distraught, when she listens to music, sings, claps her hands, and beams with joy, when she can make chicken soup and coleslaw, even if she is supervised, when she laughs at a joke, when she forgets the emotional pain experienced just moments before, when she hugs and kisses with great warmth, when we pray and she says, "I feel so peaceful that I can go to heaven right now."

So what is my responsibility for my mom's care? It is a question that I ask myself almost daily. I call frequently and visit several times a year. I talk to her caretakers. This helps me determine the level of care she needs and is receiving. I pray for peace of mind, wisdom, and healing. I know that this may come only when Mom's soul is finally free from her earthly body. I accept that we are all doing the best we can.

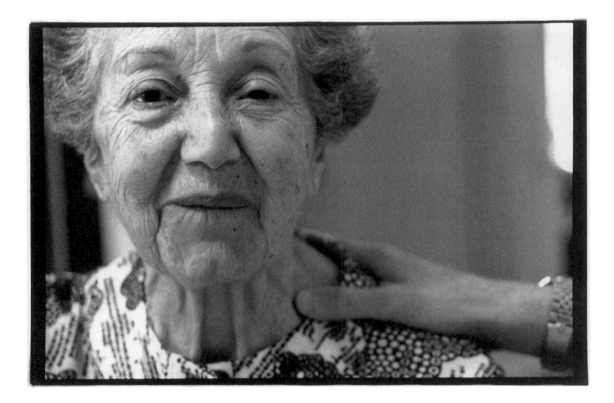

Care, compassion, and understanding combine with
the confusion, frustrations, and terrifying aspects of
this illness to bring about some semblance of order to
their lives. The family will take one day at a time,
always aware that decisions will have to be made
almost daily as Lillian's condition continues to
deteriorate.

IN JIM'S OWN WORDS

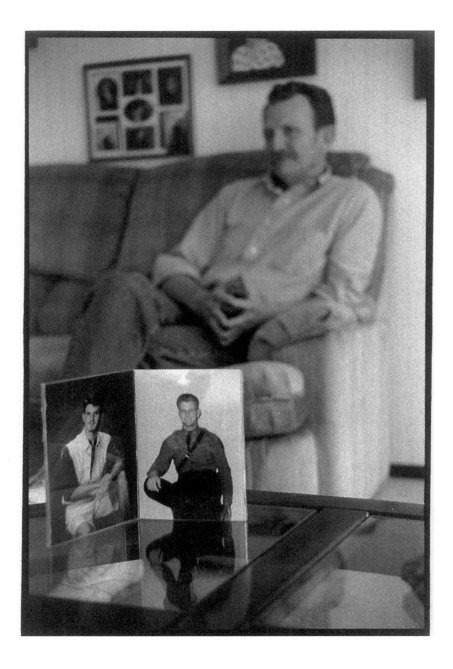

Jim Carter has early-onset Alzheimer's. At age fifty-two, he retired as a Missouri Highway Patrolman. He tells his own story.

Q:

You were telling me what it was like for you to have Alzheimer's, yesterday.

A: Oh, yesterday, yesterday.

Q: Or whenever it was.

A: The hardest thing in the world . . . it, just drove me crazy, ah, crazy.
And it was just . . . and I, ah. There's times that I didn't even know
where I was at. And that's what really gets me there. And, ah . . . now,
it's, you know, there's, there's good days and there's bad, bad days.

Q: Oh. What are the good days like?

A: The good days, it's ah. There's days that it's just like a regular roo
. . . a regular day. Sometimes. And then, and then there's days that I
don't even know what I'm doing or how I'm getting, doing things and
things like that. And that's, and that's the hardest part right there. You
get into it and it'll, it'll stop for a little while and then it'll . . . and then
it keeps on going. And it, it just drives me crazy. And it really just . . .
and like I said, ah, I said there's days that I don't, don't even know what
I'm doing . . . and that gives me the willies, you know.

Q: Oh, I can imagine.

A: Yeah.

Q: I mean, I would think it would be very scary.

A: Oh, yeah . . . and it, it . . . you know. I don't know what I'm doing. . . . As a matter of fact, when I, when I was in, in the, in the patrol . . . they, uh . . . my captain, you know . . . I was driving. And, ah, you know, the captain said, says, "Jim, I'm sorry. You've just got to go." Because I, I couldn't do it, in, in that time. And, and then, that's when I got retired.

Q: Did you know what was happening, did you know why he said that?

A: Un huh.

Q: You knew something was wrong?

A: Oh, yeah. Yeah . . .

Q: What was it like?

A: Well, the . . . well the captain, you know, h-h-he was a good old, old, guy, you know. He would do anything good for ya . . . and, ah . . . and, uh, uh . . . see now, see it's stopped now. But it'll stop every, every once in a while 'cause, it, um. But anyway, but it's, it's, ah, horrible, horrible, horrible, horrible. It's just one of those things and how I get there, I don't know. It's terrible. It's bad.

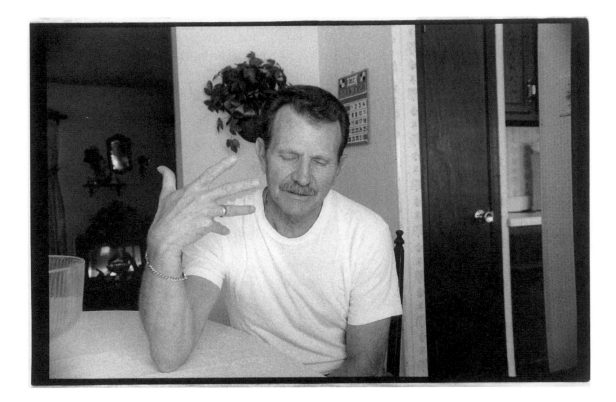

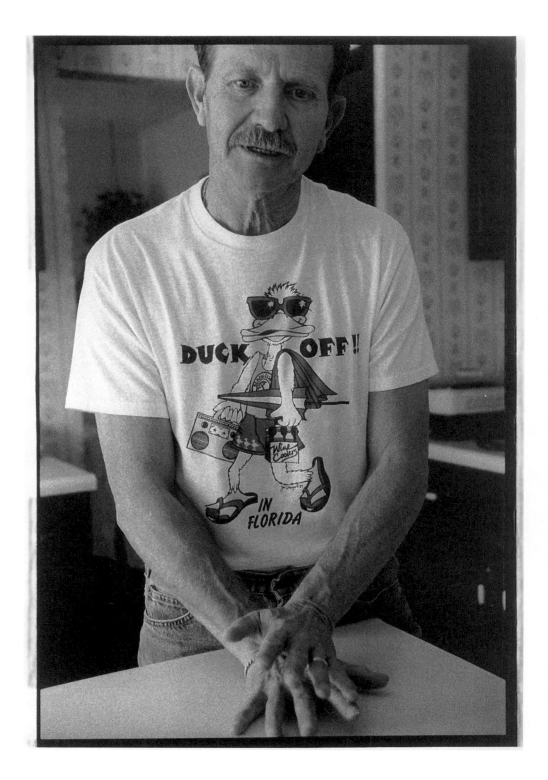

Q: What has it done to your life?

A: My life?

Q: Yes.

A: My life is something I, I could have, I could have been a, a . . . a . . . my highway patrol, ah . . . and I could have kept going, you know. But, ah, but I didn't. I couldn't do it because I, I couldn't do it before this thing. And, . . . bad, bad, bad.

Q: I would say I can imagine, but I can't imagine. It must be awful.

A: It is. And, like I said, it's, . . . there's good days and there's bad days.

Q: What is today?

A: Today is, I don't know, I don't know.

Q: You have one brother you were saying?

A: Yeah, I got one brother and he lives in, oh let's see, he lives down in ah, Cape Girardeau or somewhere down there. And he lives . . . he works in in a gin, a ginning ginny. It's a, it's a . . . do you know what a gin is?

Q: Gin?

A: A gin in ah gin?

Q: No.

A: Okay.

Q: What is it?

A: Well, it's a gin. They they ah . . . pickin' cotton.

Q: I didn't know they did that anymore.

A: Oh yeah. All they got is a great big thing to do it and it does it but back a long time ago all you do is just have to pick the cotton out, throw it out, you know.

Q: Oh.

A: Uh uh. See you played me, see, see you said something to that now or said something good to that.

Q: What do you mean?

A: What day is this . . . I don't know. Oh me, oh my.

Q: Is it a good day or a bad day?

A: Oh, it's a pretty good day today, but it has been, you know it's been out, but you know there's the good days, and it is the good days and then there's days . . . like I said I don't know what I am doing and . . . it's ah, so hard to do and like I said there's good days and there are bad days. That's what drives me sort of crazy. I shouldn't have been able to drive a long time ago. You know . . . and to the patrol, you know, and

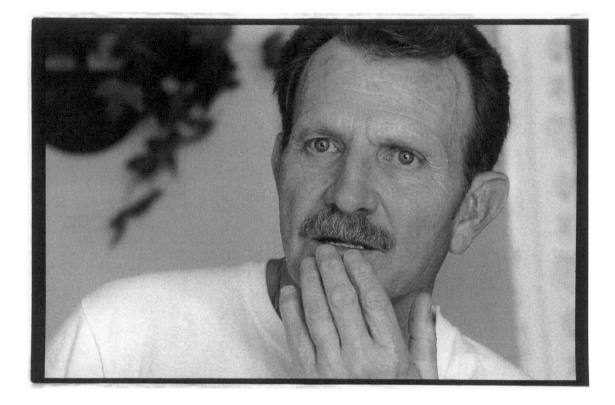

so I had a a retirement, so I had to get out. So, and, but it wasn't too bad. But like I said there's good days and there's bad days.

Q: When she [Sherry, his wife] gets home will she cook dinner? You don't cook anymore, right?

A: No. No, she's afraid that I'll burn something . . .

Q: So she gets home and then she cooks?

A: Yeah. Or either that or we'll go go down and go eat somewhere or something.

Q: Kelly [his daughter] doesn't cook?

A: Uh?

Q: Kelly doesn't cook?

A: Kelly don't cook. No.

Q: (Laughter)

A: Yeah, she does every every once in a while, every once in a while. Yeah. Kelly is a pretty good little girl . . . yeah, she's kind of goofy though.

Q: Oh?

A: Yeah, (laughter) but ah, what time is it?

Q: It's twenty after four.

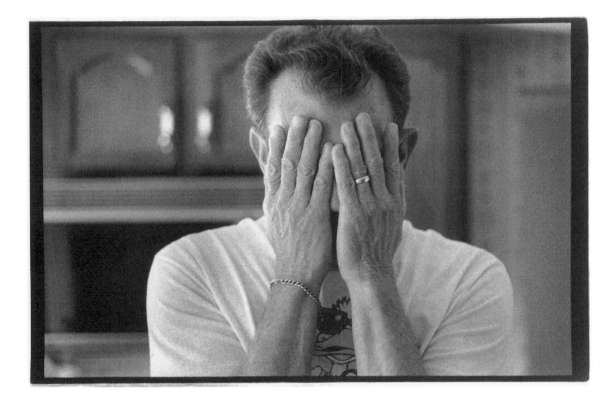

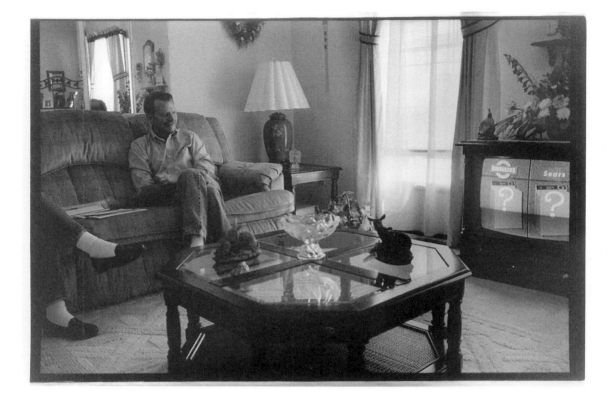

A: Oh, Sherry should be coming in pretty soon.

Q: Yes, well, if she doesn't feel well she won't need me around, so I should leave.

A: She puked her guts out last night.

Q: Oh that is terrible.

A: She was, she was sick, sick, sick.

Q: What a shame!

A: That's a nasty thing too.

Q: Oh yeah. But she was able to go to work this morning?

A: Yeah.

Q: What time does she leave? She said she works ten hours.

A: Yeah.

Q: So she must leave at four in the morning.

A: She does, she does.

Q: Amazing. I could never do that.

A: See that's that's the way, the way the patrol does that.

Q: Oh.

A: And, uh, so I done forgot what we were talking about.

Q: We were talking about getting up at four in the morning.

A: Yeah, yeah. Well, she's, I mean she does. She's done it so long it doesn't matter, you know. She gets in her car; she's gone. She's strong. She's a strong lady, I tell you.

Q: She seems to be.

A: She is. If it wasn't for her I'd probably be dead you know because I, I think that 'cause she's, she's so sweet and beautiful, just love her to death.

Q: That's nice.

A: And that's enough, that's right. Sure nuff.

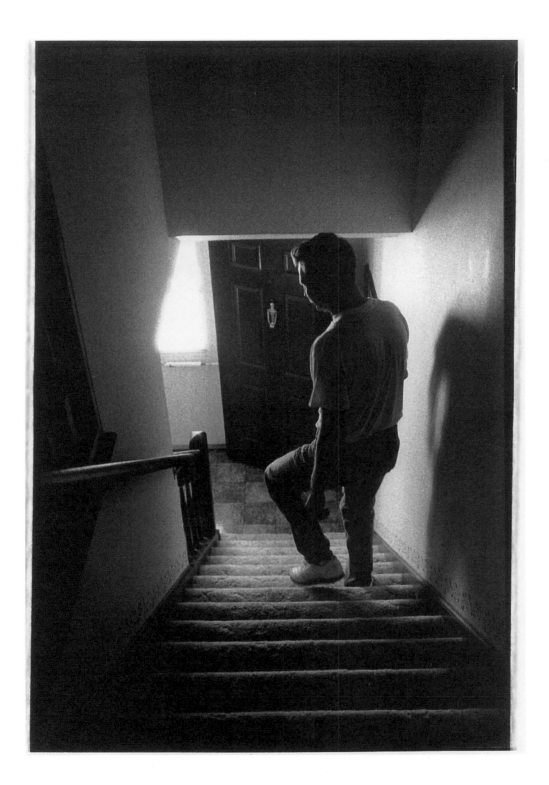

JIM'S WIFE SHERRY'S STORY

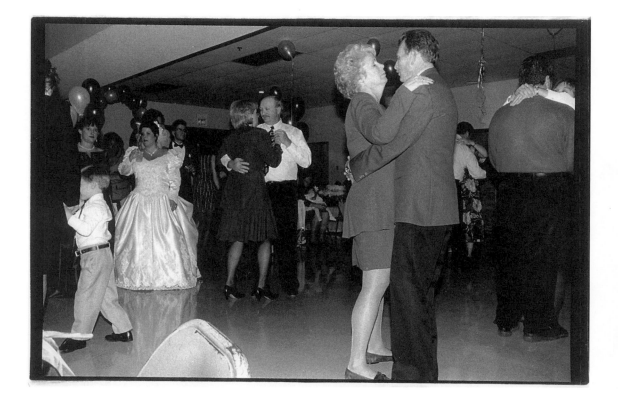

J im's boss was concerned that maybe Jim had a brain tumor. We both worked for the Missouri Highway Patrol. Jim began as a state trooper when he was eighteen years old. I followed after our marriage to work in the office.

At age fifty-two, Jim started to show signs of something not being right. For months we went to doctor after doctor. "Well, I think it's stress." "Well, I think it's nerves." "No, I think it's this." "No, I think it's that." I wish they could make the diagnosis sooner so we don't have to be shuffled around month after month. Jim had every test; that's the hard part: not knowing and feeling like, "Am I crazy? Have I lost my mind?" You think you are imagining it or there's something psychologically wrong with you. At first no one took us seriously, especially after they ruled out brain tumor and other abnormalities of the brain. They ply you with all this medicine. Prozac, then this one and then that one. He became a zombie. He couldn't function.

But he did get better and the doctor said he could go back to work. I don't know how he did it though. He was trying so hard to do his job but really couldn't. I wish they could come up with a better way to diagnose.

The last doctor we went to before we found our wonderful doctor at Washington University was a neurologist who had the worst bedside manner. He was very blunt and told us straight out that he thought Jim had Alzheimer's disease. Jim said he had thought so too, had always thought so. But I didn't; I didn't even consider it. Alzheimer's was for old people, not someone fifty-two years old!

That doctor sent us to Washington University's department for Alzheimer's and they confirmed the diagnosis. Jim kept saying he had Alzheimer's and said, "Thank God it is not a brain tumor!" The doctors there thought that was so neat; he had such a good outlook. He's had a good outlook from day one, you know. He never gets down. He gets mad at himself and he really likes to beat on himself, but he never blames anybody but himself. I guess you have to have a good attitude about it. You really do. But that is the way he has always been. He's always taken one day at a time and had a lot of faith in God.

The kids keep him going too. The kids are around all the time here. Two of our teenagers live at home. Our oldest daughter lives nearby. Our middle daughter lives here with her husband and is pregnant. So lots goes on here.

Sometimes he gets aggravated at them because they're always here, always eating. It gets old and he gets tired of it, but when you have younger people around all the time it keeps you young. Basically, you couldn't stand it if they didn't come around.

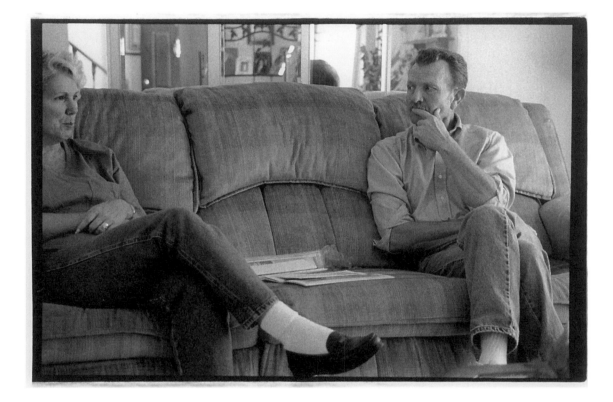

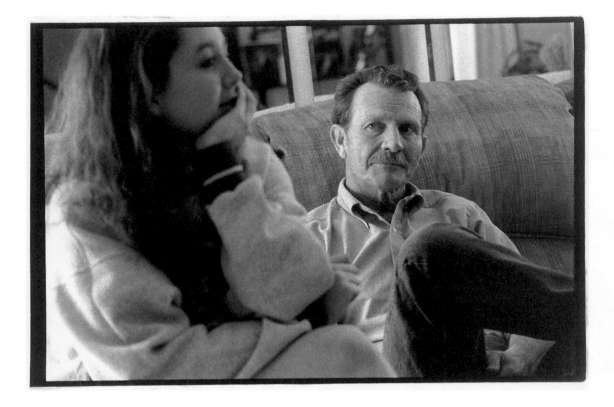

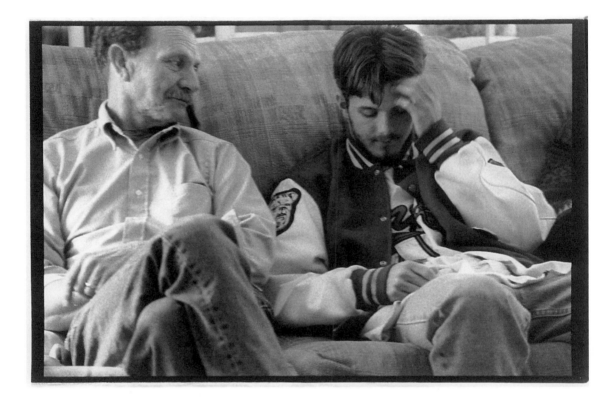

Jim is very much a part of a loving family. His son and two daughters do not dwell on his Alzheimer's; they accept him as he is.

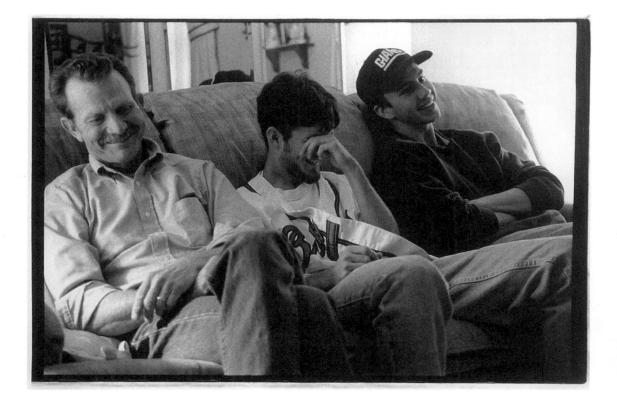

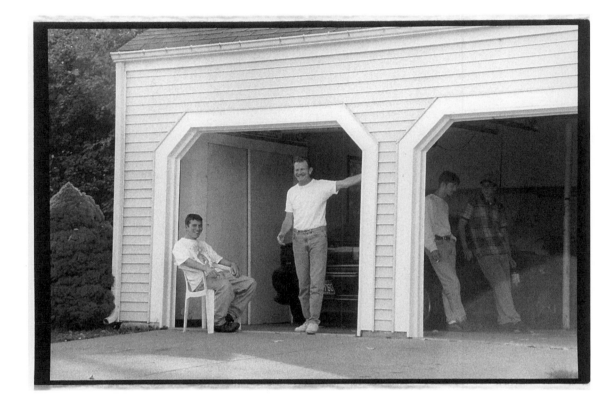

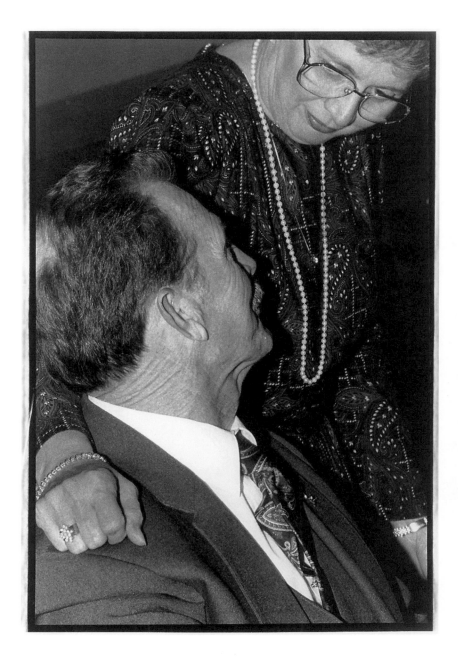

Jim can join in family celebrations almost easily. Incredible support from family and friends makes it possible.

And we're going to have a baby around here too. Jim will be playing with the baby and spoiling it. He loves babies and I really think it will be good. I will be at work during the day. My daughter will be here during the day. Her husband works at Pizza Hut. He's a delivery driver. Whatever that is.

She helps me with her father. Since she's here during the day with him it takes my mind off the fact that he is here by himself. Even though he doesn't need someone right now, he needs someone to see that he eats, because he can no longer use the stove or microwave. So it helps to have her around even if she does complain sometimes. It's not all bad, not all bad really.

Christmas is coming and it's my favorite holiday. The married kids want a mattress, of all things. How can you give someone a mattress for Christmas? I will be putting up the tree and hanging some more pictures. Of course we'll hang your pictures too.

And then there are the plaques that he got when he retired. When you retire, they give you your uniform. They gave Jim a party and the colonel comes down and presents it to you. He has his old license plate, the one he had on patrol. It has his number and "HP" behind it. It's a regular Highway Patrol plate. His number was 221. Our son wants to join the Highway Patrol. We are very proud of him.

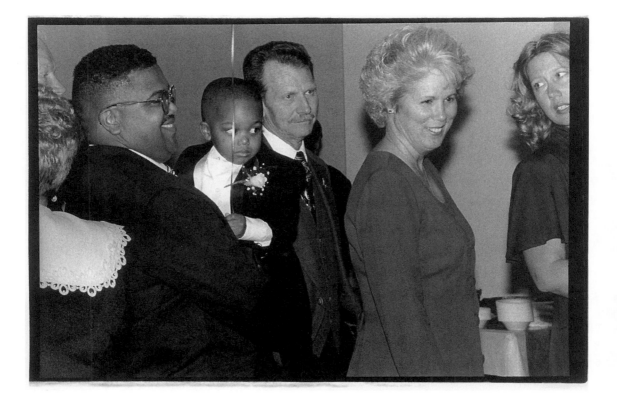

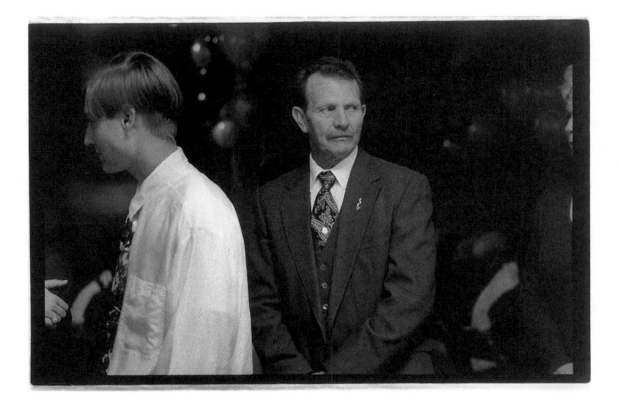

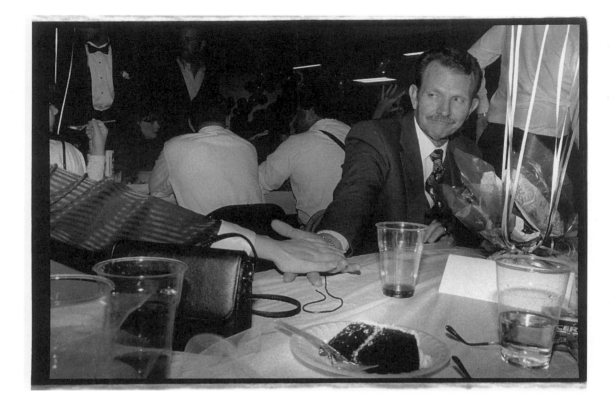

They thought Alzheimer's was for old people. But Jim knew he had Alzheimer's; he just knew it.

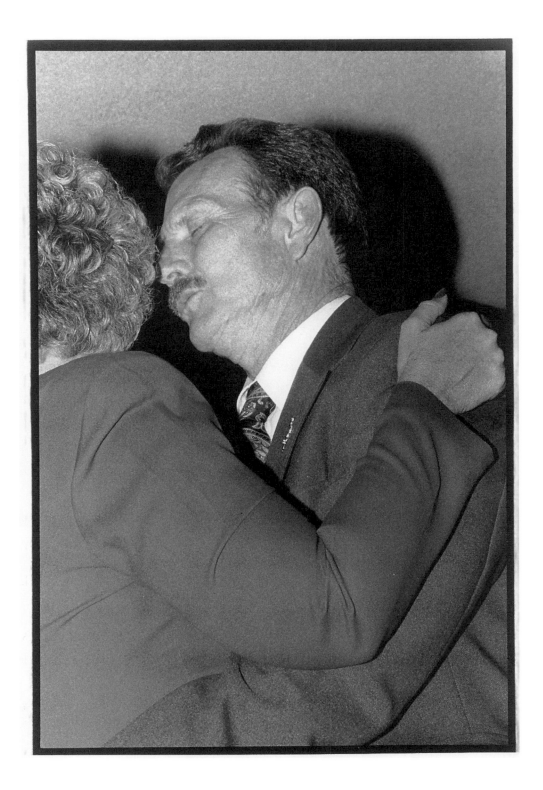

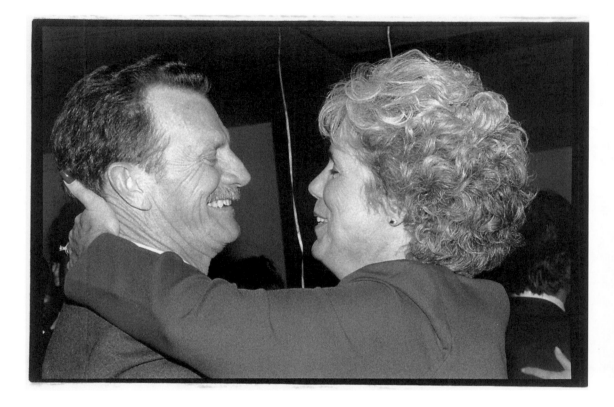

*Alzheimer's or no Alzheimer's, Jim and Sherry
Carter are still in love.*

We got involved with the Alzheimer's Association. We first got started going to a group called Project Self-Esteem for Early Onset people; it was for the patient and the caregiver. While I was in a meeting, he was in a meeting. They had a support group, and we had a support group. But when the project was over there wasn't anything more for him to do. There's a support group on every corner for the caregiver but none for the patient. We enjoyed going together. It's discouraging because there's nothing out there for him. They say he can go to day-care. But who wants to go to day-care when you're only fifty-four years old? He's too young.

I thought about starting a group myself for patients, and I think I could help someone in my shoes as a caregiver. But I wouldn't know how to deal with anybody other than him, I don't think. Sometimes they get on my nerves. I'm so used to his little ways, but I don't think I have enough patience for someone else. I think in order to deal with a patient you need to be a professional.

One group wanted to start a social hour every Sunday. I suggested dancing, but somebody said, "But some are old people." And I said, "You'd be surprised." And music is so important too. There will be a cost involved, which worries me. We can afford it but many can't. I don't know how it's going to work.

Day-care is something that people need for something to do. But Jim is still active enough to where he can keep himself busy. And with the kids being here I don't see the need for it. If he wanted to go, fine, but I don't see it as anything I want him to do right now. I don't think there's any need unless you're feeling bored at home and you have nothing to do and you're upset about being home a lot. Or if the family just couldn't stand them at home. That's not us.

Jean's Story

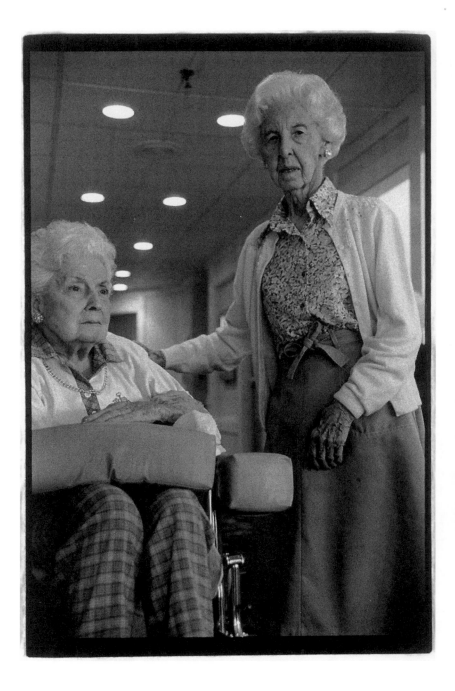

Louise Johnson, ninety, and Lina Whitmire, ninety-one, have been best friends for seventy years. They are now roommates in a nursing home. They both have Alzheimer's disease. Louise's daughter, Jean, tells their story.

My husband, Art, and I had been living in Seattle when we first suspected something was wrong with Mother. We had returned to St. Louis, where I grew up, for Christmas. When we told Mother that we would be coming, she began to plan a number of activities. She was very social. She loved company. She loved to entertain. Christmas was always a wonderful time in her home even though I was an only child. When we arrived in St. Louis, both Art and I were very aware that there was something wrong. Mother's personality seemed to be changing; her values seemed to be changing, and oftentimes the things she said were not completely true. Instead of staying two weeks as we had planned, we stayed four months.

During that time I saw Mother age, and I felt uncomfortable that she was living alone. We went back to Seattle. We sold our home and we moved to St. Louis. Mother insisted that we live with her. We wanted our own house, but I was the only child; whatever was my mother's was mine, didn't I realize that? Whenever we would talk about moving, Mother would say, "I am not going to leave this house. I love this house." Art and I realized that she was not going to leave and that we were going to be staying right there.

We completely remodeled the kitchen because Art is quite a gourmet. Until this day I can see Mother washing the dishes. She would open a drawer and the drawer she opened was not the drawer that the object belonged in. She would look up at me and say, "I always knew where everything in this kitchen went and now you have changed it and I don't know where anything goes." I would laugh and say, "Well, you will learn in due time." But due time never came. Slowly but surely I saw that she would find excuses for not coming into the kitchen. I look back now and realize why she couldn't find where things were supposed to go. I should have been tipped off that she was a wonderful actress and as time went on I found out what an excellent actress she really was. It is difficult for me to think of everything that happened and the sequence in which it happened because I didn't keep a journal. I'm sorry I didn't, because there were so many things I thought I would never forget, but the mind erases everything very, very quickly and I guess that too is very, very fortunate for all of us.

Mother belonged to various organizations and she loved to play bridge. That was always a big part of her life. She would get up, get dressed, and off to lunch she would go and play cards in the afternoon. Her friends started calling me intimating that Mother was having a little difficulty playing cards or Mother's personality was changing or Mother had said something to someone that was most unlike my mother. One friend began, "Jean, I don't know how to tell you but

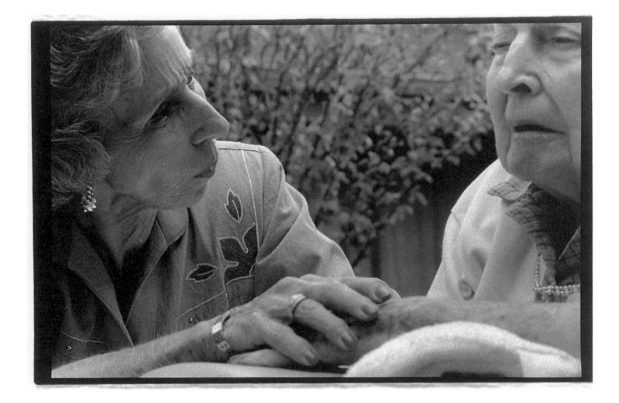

One-way conversations help Jean keep whatever is left of her relationship with her mother. She talks to her mother as she did before her mother's illness, as if Louise can still understand, care, and want to know about her daughter's daily life.

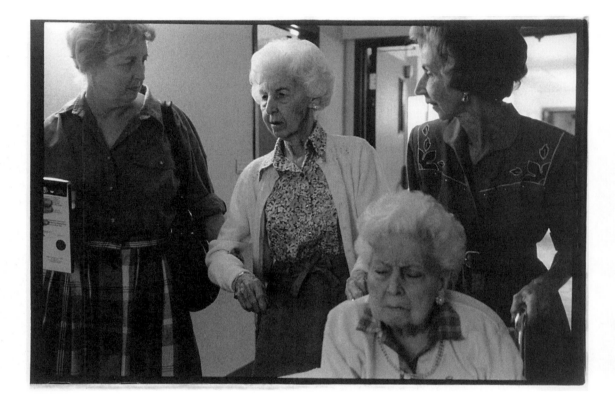

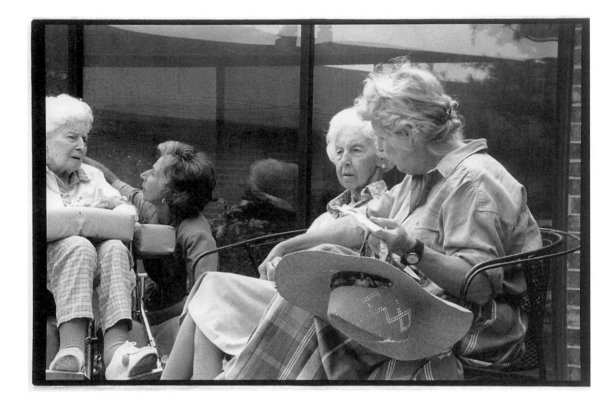

Two sets of friends. The daughters have been friends since childhood, the mothers, friends since early in their marriages. They continue to share experiences.

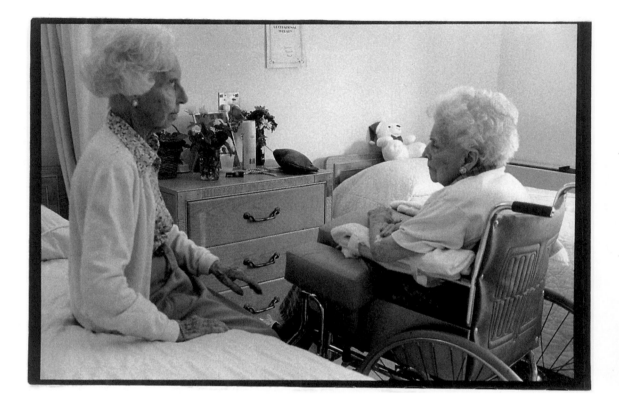

Louise is in the last stage of the disease. Lina still recognizes her daughter, Whitney, and makes attempts to communicate with Louise.

today while we were playing cards, your mother became so upset that she threw all the cards to the floor and said, 'I am not going to play this damn game again.' " The other ladies she was playing with tried to change the subject but to no avail; the game was over. After the guests had left her home, the hostess realized that the napkin where my mother had been sitting was not there. She called, embarrassed, and asked, "Jean, by any chance would your mother have taken my table napkin? I don't seem to have it and I don't know where it might be." I told her that I would check and went to my mother's purse. Sure enough, there was the napkin. I phoned the lady back and I said yes, I had found the napkin and I would return it to her. In the meantime, I did launder it.

We would take Mother to a restaurant for dinner and in a short time we had a wonderful assortment of napkins. Unfortunately, none of them matched anything we had. Well, things seemed to go from bad to worse and we finally said we had to do something, but we did not know what. One day Art was reading an article about a disease called Alzheimer's. There was a number in Chicago for information. Really, I think that was the first time I had ever heard that name. I read the information that they sent us, and the more I read I realized what was wrong with my mother.

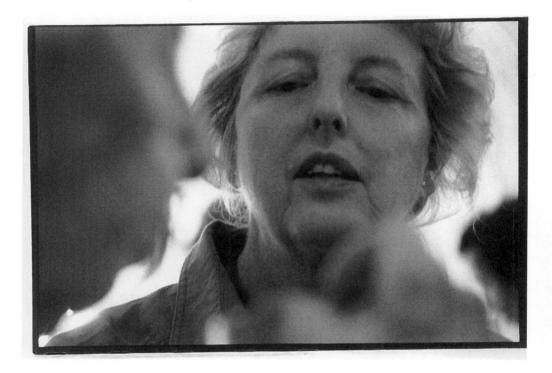

Lina lived with her daughter until the disease could no longer be contained. Whitney was a single caregiver. Her brother and sister gave little help, and she neglected a thriving business that was left to dissolve. Whitney gave up a lot to care for her mother and now experiences many periods of rage, anger, and frustration.

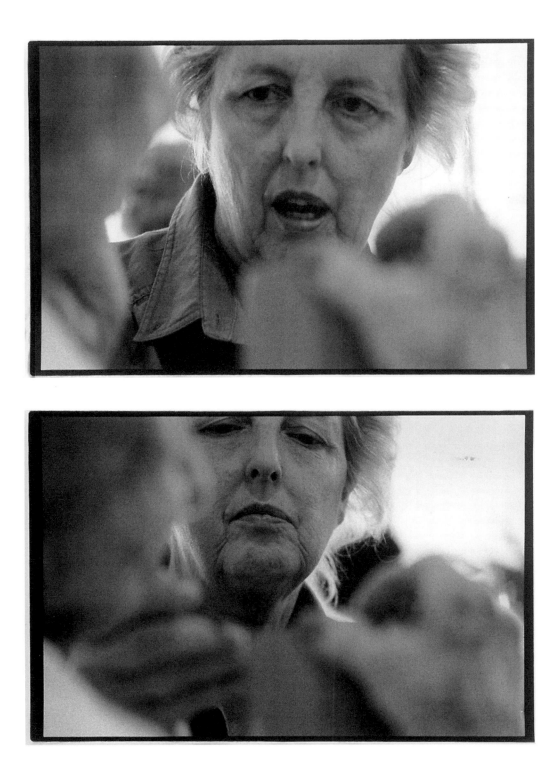

After many calls and a lot of conversation, we ended up with a doctor who specialized in geriatrics. He examined my mother several times in his office and finally suggested that she have a complete evaluation. I remember the day they were doing the memory part of the evaluation. Mother was to be there at 8:30 in the morning and she would not be finished until after 5:00 in the afternoon. When we went to pick her up for lunch the team that had been working with her took us aside and said that there was no reason to continue with the tests. I was in shock. I was told that my mother was very confused and they had done as much as they could possibly do and could do no more for her. The testing would be of no value from this point on.

Six weeks later the doctor gave us the diagnosis of probable Alzheimer's disease and said that we might expect Mother to live another five to eight years and that we should consider a nursing home. I was absolutely devastated that he could even say such a thing. The three of us went home, and I completely dismissed the idea of nursing homes from my mind because certainly she was not that sick and certainly it was not very demanding of me to take care of her. But as the months passed I realized that it was very difficult. My mother would awaken at 2:00 A.M. and I would be awakened by the light in her bedroom. I would find her fully dressed, even with hat and gloves, sitting

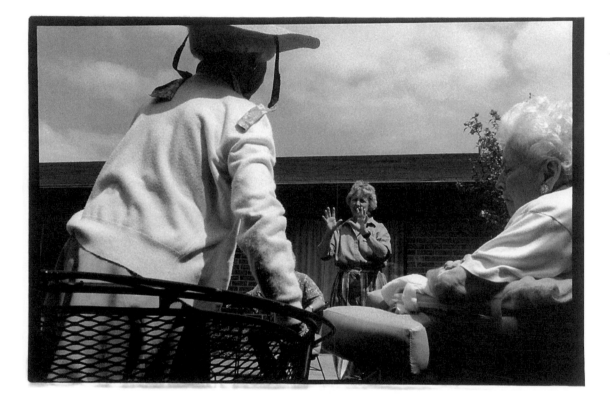

Self-control, once taken for granted, is now a conscious, constant daily struggle.

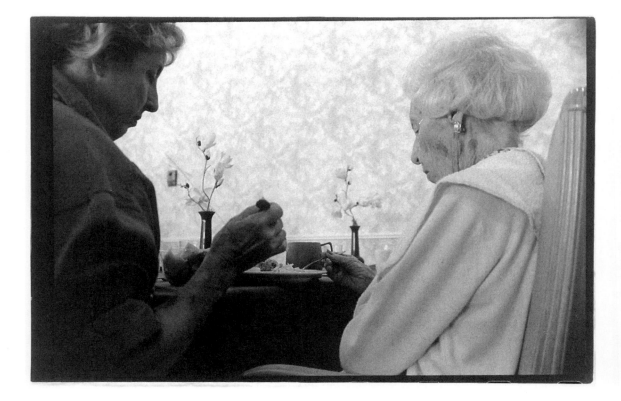

*The nursing home has relieved the daughters of
constant daily care, of the anticipation of coming
home to chaos. Relief is mingled with grief.*

in a chair. I would say, "Mom, what are you doing up? It's two o'clock in the morning." She would say, "I am ready to go. Why aren't you ready to go?" I tried to explain but I felt as if I were speaking to a child. Maybe that was a good way to handle it. As I look back now it probably was a better way to handle it than I realized. I eventually put her back in bed.

It did not take me long to realize that she was not taking baths and it was up to me to see that she was bathed. This was a difficult thing to do, because my mother is a very private person and I don't know that I have ever seen her without her clothes on. Suddenly, I was in the bathroom with her and I was giving her a bath. I was helping her dress. She was having difficulty putting clothes on in the proper order. For quite a while she was determined that she would wear at least three pair of stockings, maybe four. She did not want anyone to see her legs. I thought the color of the hose was all wrong. It was not long before she was having difficulty combing her hair, and she had always taken great pride in her hair. She had beautiful hair and her hair was never out of place. I suddenly became, not only the person who bathed my mother and dressed my mother, but also her beautician seven days a week. I did not mind but I knew I could not do it the way it should be done and this bothered me.

My mother continued to go to her bridge club, which she really shouldn't have done, but the ladies of the bridge club were so dear, so thoughtful. They would not offend her by telling her not to come, and I guess we were wrong in allowing her to go. She continued to drive, but she began coming home later and later. One afternoon, after calling the other women in the club in a vain effort to locate Mother, I started making excuses for her. I didn't want my mother's friends to know how concerned I really was about her. Then panic set in and I called the police.

They assured me they would find her. For the next four hours, many thoughts went through my mind. I thought of all the things that were happening in St. Louis and I wondered about her safety. About midnight we got a call from the sheriff's office in a town seventy-five miles from us. They had Mother. She had been picked up driving on the shoulder of the road very, very slowly. We explained that we would be there as soon as we could get there. We hopped in the car. We drove out, and when we arrived at the sheriff's office, my mother was her true social, Southern-belle self. She was entertaining the police and the sheriff. They were all sitting around simply mesmerized by her. I almost expected her to be licking an ice cream cone.

The next morning we suggested to her that perhaps it would be best for her not to drive, that what had happened last night was very

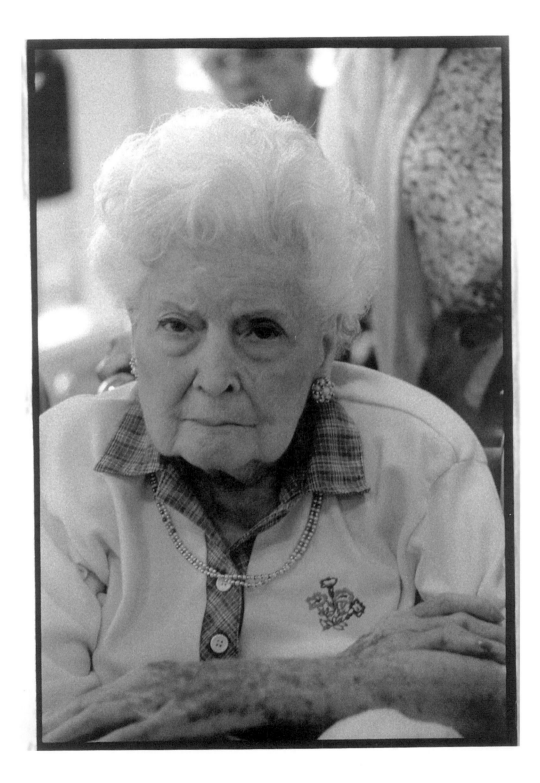

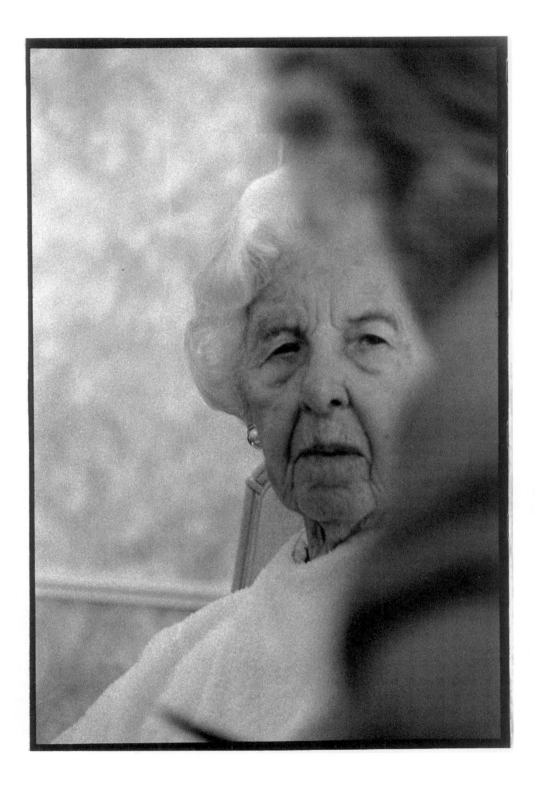

hard for us to handle. We were concerned for her safety. But she assured us that she would be all right and she was going to continue to drive! It wasn't whether we wanted her to or not, she was just going to continue to drive. For the next few weeks, whenever she got in the car, I would always find a reason why I had to go wherever she was going. But you know, eventually that wears kind of thin and you become very lax; I certainly did. After six months, she was back playing bridge at friends' homes. And again one day she did not return home for many hours.

We waited again before calling the police but then had to. By this time we felt like old friends; they were very kind as they had been the first time. They reassured us that they would find my mother. That night it took them a lot longer. It was 2:00 A.M. when I got the call. The police had located my mother. She was driving in circles on a parking lot.

The next morning I told her she was not going to drive any more. She cried for the next two weeks. We were taking her last bit of independence. She never had an accident, she never had a ticket, and how could we do this to her? For two weeks she sat in the chair and cried. I never felt so sorry for anybody in my life. I could do nothing, because I could not say, "Mom, you can drive," because I knew we

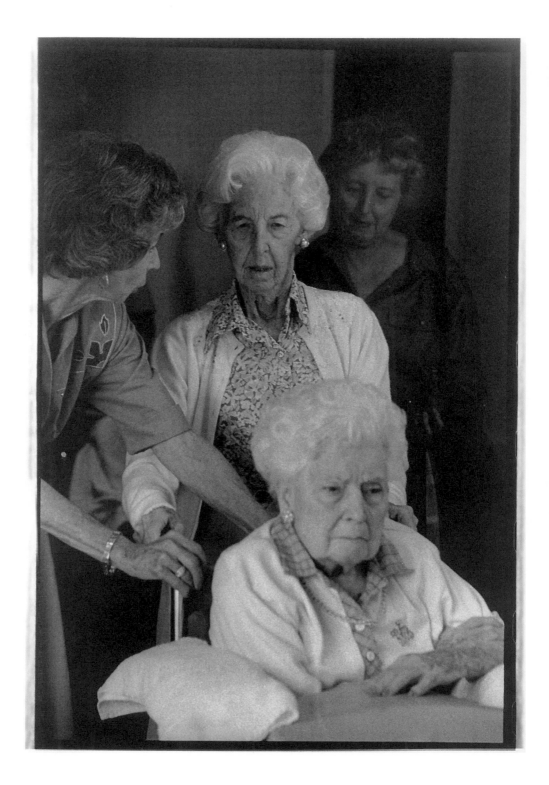

could not go through that again. Finally, I guess Art just felt he had to say something, and he said, "Mom, I'll tell you what. You give us twenty-four hours and we'll pack our things and we will leave, and once we are out of town you can drive, but at least we won't know about it and we won't worry about you." They were magical words. She never spoke of driving again to us. Now she told her friends that we would not let her drive and that she did not know why, but she would not talk to us about it.

She began to tell some rather unbelievable stories. We were having dinner in a new restaurant and she told us that she had been to this restaurant for lunch that day. She told us all about the people who had been there for lunch, although none of us had ever been to that restaurant before. We realized that we just let her say whatever she wanted to because she probably did not realize what in the world she was saying.

Throughout, Art has been unbelievable. I have never known anybody so unselfish. He has done things for my mother that I would not even have thought about. He has never been cross with her. He has always been so kind and so gentle and so good. He will never know how much I appreciate what he has done. I don't know if I could do all that he has done for my mother.

We went back to the doctor to see about a new test drug that we heard about. The doctor asked if I had made any decisions about a nursing home. I said no, I saw no reason to. He then suggested an adult day-care situation. This would give us some respite time and time alone for my husband and me. I didn't think too much about it at first, but then I thought about it more, and I realized that mother was becoming dependent upon me for all her activities and this would be a good idea. I selected a day-care, and I must tell you that for the next year my mother would not tell you that she enjoyed it, but I know that she did. We explained where she would be going and this did not seem to bother her too much. The first few times we went, she was a little reluctant to get out of the car, but she would and she would go in. But after a few times, when I drove her to the parking lot of the day-care she would look at me and say, "I am not going in." My mother really didn't know who I was and yet she knew she was not going into the day-care. We did have a hard time getting her to go, and it took two of us to get her out of the car.

It was not too long before we realized that my mother had a boyfriend. We just thought that this was wonderful. It started out that he and my mother would dance together when the day-care had some ballroom dancing. And before long they were sitting next to each

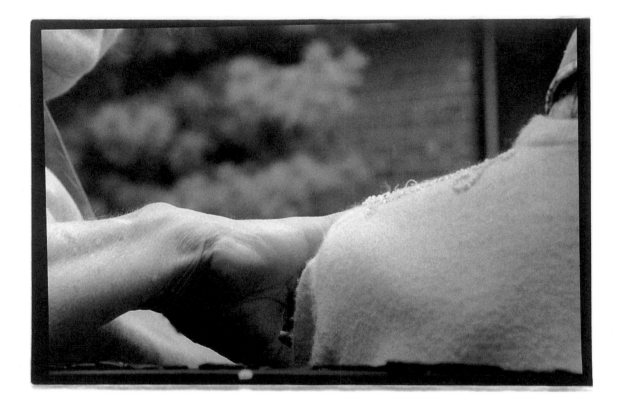

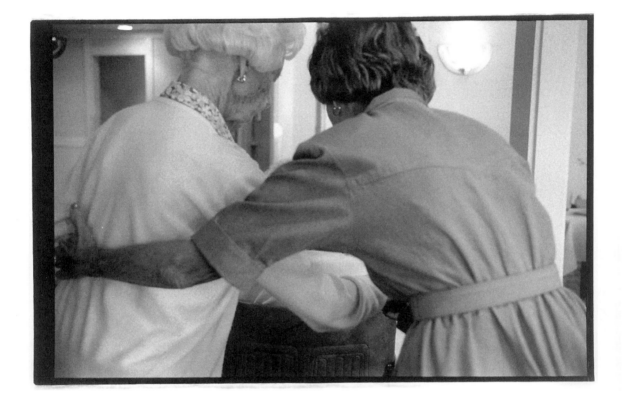

other, and before too long he would wait at the door for my mother to arrive. This man was married; he had a wife! The staff assured me that the wife knew all about it, and it did not really make any difference because for a few hours these two people had someone that they were comfortable with and they could let all their pretenses of coping with the world slip by.

We drove my mother forty miles to this day-care. We started out three days a week, but before you knew it, it developed into four and then it was five. Her days were filled with pleasurable activities. They had parties. They went on trips, and Mother seemed to enjoy herself. I was told at the end of the year that my mother had been there, that I should consider a vacation. I didn't accept that too well because I had a great responsibility. I was taking care of my mother and I did not have time to take care of myself and my husband. I guess I had completely forgotten about Art. I was so involved with my mother and my fears for her, I dismissed it from my mind, but they insisted. I had been looking at nursing homes, and I suddenly thought, "Okay. I will call the nursing home and see if they can take my mother for a month and we will take a vacation. Maybe we won't be gone a whole month, but we will tell them that we will have my mother stay a month. We'll take a vacation and when we come back, my mother will come back home.

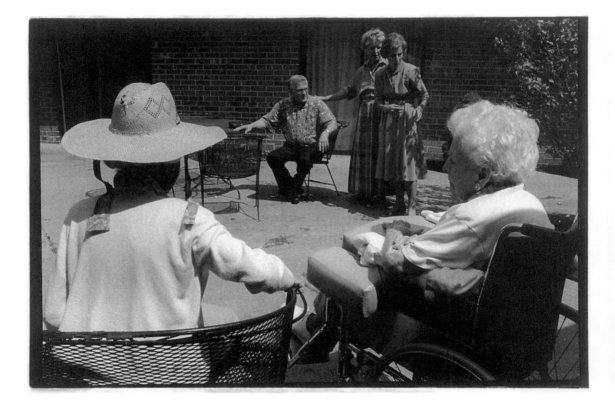

Art, Jean's husband, has been close to his mother-in-law throughout his marriage. His continuous loving support of his wife and her mother has helped to sustain the family.

We will all live happily together again. She will continue going to day-care just as we had done for the past year." I made the call and was numb.

I did explain to her about the nursing home and that we would return soon. I tried to be as honest about the whole situation as I could possibly be. Then of course, Art and I had to scurry around to see what we were going to do while my mother was in the nursing home. We took my mother to the home and we all had lunch together. After lunch Mother was invited to the card club. She did not seem to care whether we were there or not.

I went back the next day because I knew that my mother would not be able to dress herself, and I really did not know that aides dressed them or bathed them. I was very ignorant about nursing homes, and much to my surprise, when I got there my mother looked very nice. Her hair was combed and she had on a nice-looking outfit and she seemed to be very content. I breathed another sigh of relief, and I thought, "Oh boy, this isn't going to be so bad after all." I finally explained to her that we would be going away the next day and she would not be seeing us for a while. I was not going to call her but I would write her postcards while we were away.

Art and I were gone about two weeks and went straight to the

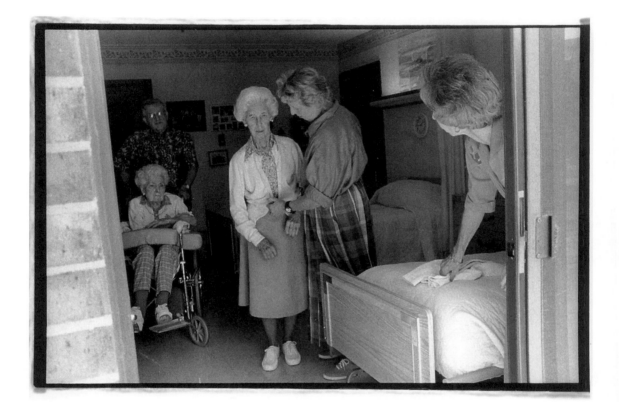

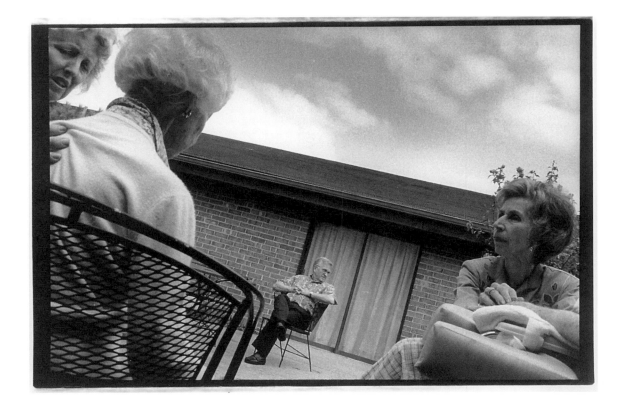

The friends support each other; little did they suspect that their lifelong togetherness would help them through this crisis.

nursing home when we arrived home. My mother was in the beauty shop. We stood at the door, we smiled, we said hello, and my mother looked up and I knew then what I had known for so long, that my mother did not even know who I was. She had not seen me. I had been erased out of her mind. I went over, I kissed her and said, "Oh, how good it is to see you." There was no response whatsoever. The tears rolled down my face and I said, "Art, this is where my mother belongs. She doesn't belong at home with us. She will be better cared for here than any place else."

The first spring my mother was in the home, I went to visit her often, but I was very concerned about having her come back to her house for a visit. Mother's Day would be the day she would return for that visit. We invited Lina Whitmire and her daughter, Whitney. Lina had been a very old and dear friend of hers and they would be with us for Mother's Day dinner. Whitney would pick up Mother. I remember when Whitney drove up to the front of the house. I went out to the door to greet them. I went out to help Mother out of the car, and she looked at me and said, "Who's house is this?" My mother had built that house about thirty years before, had lived in that house for thirty years. She didn't seem very comfortable that day, and shortly after we ate, she looked up and said, "I want to go home." So, again, this was reconfirmed that the nursing home had become her home and her life, and every-thing she knew had been erased and now her life was in the nursing home. I cry when I think about it. I wonder how anything could be so erased, and yet I cannot dwell upon it, I have to go forward.

My mother was spending more and more time in bed and be-coming more and more isolated. One day Whitney called and asked, "What would you think about our mothers rooming together in the nurs-ing home?" Whitney's mother had been diagnosed with Alzheimer's, and after many years of struggling to keep her in her own home, Whitney had decided too that the time had come for nursing home care. I thought about it a minute. "Well, Whitney, you know my mother no longer speaks and Mother spends most of her days in bed, but if you think it wouldn't bother your mother, I think it would be fine." So today Lina and Louise are roommates together; they have been friends for seventy years.

They met each other when they first moved to St. Louis. Through those seventy years they've had some very, very happy times; they've had some very sad times. Lina has three children, a son and two daughters. My mother has only one. My father passed away at age fifty. He was extremely young and the Whitmires were so thoughtful of my mother and my father during his lifetime. In the last stages of my father's illness, Dr. Whitmire used to drive by the house and if he saw my father

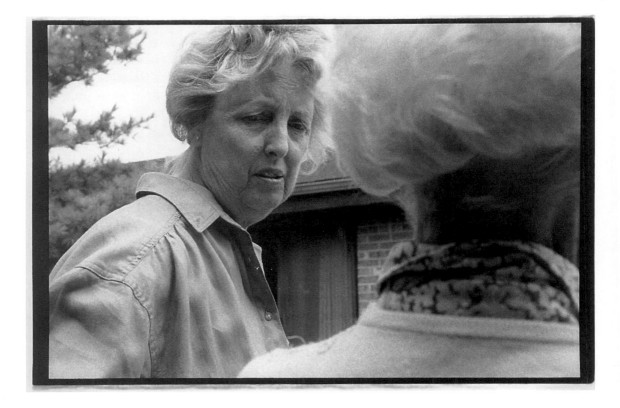

A daughter sees a relationship dissolving. Parent and child come full circle.

sitting on the porch, he would come in just to say hello. He would stay for maybe five or ten minutes and then he would be on his way. His acts of friendship and Lina's acts of friendship and kindness during my father's illness will never be forgotten. After my father passed away, Lina and her husband continued to be very supportive of my mother. They included my mother in an evening group that they participated in. They did many things for my mother, and I think I thanked them more than once for all they had done for her through the years.

Unfortunately, Dr. Whitmire had a very tragic illness. Mother tried to be very supportive to Lina during this time. After Dr. Whitmire's death, I think the two women again made a tight bond of friendship. They had both lost their husbands; they had married children. Whitney was living away from St. Louis, as I was. So many similarities through their lives—and now to think they are together. I know little that I can say except their friendship runs very, very deep and the circle is very small.

I oftentimes wonder if my mother recognizes Lina because, as I said, my mother does not speak. Lina tells me that she has wonderful visits with my mother, and I think this is grand that she thinks she does. But one day recently, Lina looked at me and she pointed to my mother and she shook her head and said, "Bad." I don't know if she meant my mother is helpless bad, or what she saw was bad. I did not pursue it. I tried to change the subject because Lina is still very rational. She can carry on a conversation, and you can swing the subjects around and talk about happy things.

You know, when I go to the nursing home I sit and talk to my mother. I tell her what I did today, or what I did yesterday. I talk about when the seasons change, getting the clothes out of the closet, the new ones in, and going through my old clothes. I often laugh and say, "Boy, that basket of mending is really getting kind of big." She used to love to knit and I do not know how to sew a stitch.

I sometimes wonder if she understands what I am talking about, but I know this, that I am going to keep on visiting her even though it is a one-sided visit. As long as my mother is in that bed, I will go to that home; I will visit with her and I will hold her hand and I will look into her eyes and I will tell her how much I love her and what a good mother she has been and how sorry I am that I did not have a child that I could pass on some of the strength and courage she has passed on to me. I know without that strength I could not make it this far. I love her dearly; I guess you could say this is unconditional love. I don't think anyone deserves this kind of illness. It affects us all. Someone once said it is a very long good-bye. I think it is. It is the longest good-bye I will ever have to say.

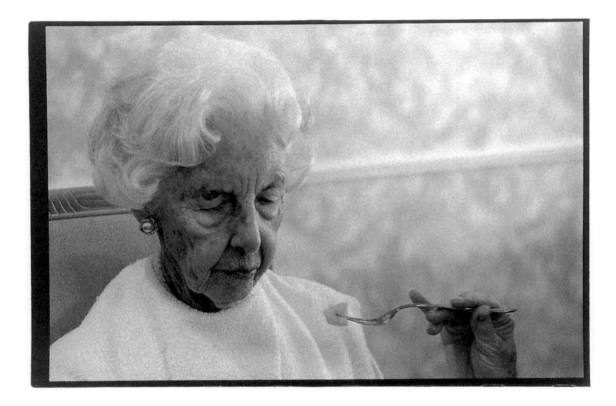

Waiting for death is more intense than ever before in life. Release now engenders hope; hope takes on a whole new meaning.

USEFUL ORGANIZATIONS

Resources for Families Dealing with Alzheimer's Disease

A list of addresses and telephone numbers for the approximately 225 regional offices of the Alzheimer's Association is available through the national headquarters in Chicago.

Alzheimer's Association, National Headquarters
919 N. Michigan Avenue, Suite 1000
Chicago, IL 60611
(800) 272-3900 (outside Ill.)
(800) 572-6037 (in Ill.)
(312) 853-3060
http://www.alz.org

Alzheimer's Association, Los Angeles Chapter
5900 Wilshire Boulevard
Los Angeles, CA 90036
(800) 660-1993
(213) 938-3379

Alzheimer's Association, Greater Phoenix Chapter
1028 E. McDowell Avenue
Phoenix, AZ 85006
(800) 392-0022
(602) 528-0545

Alzheimer's Association, Greater San Francisco Chapter
330 Distel Circle
Los Altos, CA 94002
(800) 660-1993
(415) 962-8111

Alzheimer's Association, Greater Miami Chapter
11900 Biscayne Boulevard
Miami, FL 33181
(305) 891-6228

Alzheimer's Association, New York City Chapter
420 Lexington Avenue
New York, NY 10170
(212) 983-0070

Alzheimer's Association, Philadelphia Chapter
100 N. 17th Street
Philadelphia, PA 19103
(800) 559-0404
(215) 568-6430

Alzheimer's Association, St. Louis Chapter
9374 Olive Blvd.
St. Louis, MO 63132-3214
(800) 980-9080
(314) 432-3422

General Information on the Issues of Aging

American Association of Retired Persons
601 E Street NW
Washington, DC 20049
(202) 434-2277

National Association of Area Agencies on Aging
1112 16th Street NW, Suite 100
Washington, DC 20036
(202) 296-8130

Resources for Adult Children of Aging Parents

Aging Network Services
4400 East-West Highway, Suite 907
Bethesda, MD 20814
(301) 657-4329

Children of Aging Parents
Woodbourne Office Campus, Suite 302A
1609 Woodbourne Road
Levittown, PA 19057
(215) 945-6900

National Association of Private Geriatric Care Managers
655 N. Alvernon Way, Suite 108
Tucson, AZ 85711
(602) 881-8008

General Information on Legal and Financial Issues

National Academy of Elder Law Attorneys, Inc.
655 N. Alvernon Way, Suite 108
Tucson, AZ 85711
(602) 881-4005

National Citizens' Coalition for Nursing Home Reform
1224 M Street NW, Suite 301
Washington, DC 20005
(202) 393-2018

National Hospice Organization
1901 N. Moore Street, Suite 901
Arlington, VA 22209
(800) 658-8898
(703) 243-5900

SUGGESTED RESOURCES

Readings

Alzheimer's Association. *Family Guide: For Alzheimer Care in Residential Settings.* Chicago, Ill.: Alzheimer's Disease and Related Disorders Association, 1992.

———.*Respite Care Guide.* Chicago, Ill.: Alzheimer's Disease and Related Disorders Association, 1995.

———.*Terms and Tips: An Alzheimer Care Handbook.* Chicago, Ill.: Alzheimer's Disease and Related Disorders Association, 1995.

Coughlin, Patricia. *Facing Alzheimer's: Family Caregivers Speak.* New York: Ballantine Books, 1993.

Fox, P. "From Senility to Alzheimer's Disease: The Rise of the Alzheimer's Disease Movement." *Milbank Quarterly* 67, no. 1 (1989): 58–102.

Gray, David Dodson. *I Want to Remember: A Son's Reflection on His Mother's Alzheimer Journey.* Wellesley, Mass.: Roundtable Press, 1993.

Guthrie, D. *Grandpa Doesn't Know It's Me.* New York: Human Sciences Press, 1986.

Heath, A. *Long-Distance Caregiving: A Survival Guide for Faraway Caregivers.* Lakewood, Colo.: American Source Books, 1993.

Horowitz, K. E., and D. M. Lanes. *Witness to Illness: Strategies for Caregiving and Coping.* Reading, Mass.: Addison-Wesley, 1992.

Journeyworks Publishing. *Caring for a Person with Memory Loss and Confusion.* Santa Cruz, Calif.: Journeyworks Publishing, 1995.

Jury, M., and D. Jury. *Gramps: Photographs.* New York: Grossman, 1976.

Karr, K. L. *Taking Time for Me: How Caregivers Can Effectively Deal with Stress.* Buffalo, N.Y.: Prometheus Books, 1992.

Lyman, K. A. *Day In, Day Out with Alzheimer's: Stress in Caregiving Relationships.* Philadelphia, Pa.: Temple University Press, 1993.

Mace, Nancy L., and Peter V. Rabins. *The Thirty-Six Hour Day*. New York: Warner Books, 1981.

Millard, Mary Ann. *If You Don't Laugh, You'll Cry*. San Bernadino, Calif.: Western Graphics, 1994.

Oliver, R., and F. A. Bock. *Coping with Alzheimer's: A Caregiver's Emotional Survival Guide*. New York: Dodd, Mead, 1987.

Pollen, Daniel A. *Hannah's Heirs: The Quest for the Genetic Origins of Alzheimer's Disease*. New York: Oxford University Press, 1993.

Powell, Lenore, and Katie Courtice. *Alzheimer's Disease: A Guide for Families*. Reading, Mass.: Addison-Wesley, 1994.

Pritkin, E., and T. Reece. *Parentcare Survival Guide: Helping Your Folks Through the Not-So-Golden Years*. Hauppage, N.Y.: Barron's, 1993.

Roberts, Jeanne D. *Taking Care of Caregivers: For Families and Others Who Care for People with Alzheimer's Disease and Other Forms of Dementia*. Palo Alto and Emeryville, Calif.: Bull Publishing, 1991.

Sheridan, Carmel. *Failure-Free Activities for the Alzheimer Patient: A Guidebook for Caregivers*. San Francisco, Calif.: Cottage Books, 1987.

Simpson, Carol. *At the Heart of Alzheimer's*. Silver Springs, Md.: Manor HealthCare Corp., 1996.

Smith, Kerri. *Caring for Your Aging Parents: A Sourcebook of Timesaving Techniques and Tips*. Lakewood, Colo.: American Source Books, 1992.

Spohr, B., and J. Bullard. *To Hold a Falling Star: Living at Home with Alzheimer's*. Stanford, Conn.: Longmeadow Press, 1990.

Starkman, Elaine Marcus. *Learning to Sit in Silence: A Journal of Caretaking*. Watsonville, Calif: Papier-Mache Press, 1992.

Wright, Lore K. *Alzheimer's Disease and Marriage*. Newbury Park, Calif.: Sage Publishing, 1993.

Videos

"Complaints of a Dutiful Daughter." 44 min., 1994.
> Women Make Movies
> 462 Broadway, 5th Floor
> New York, NY 10013
> (212) 925-0606

"Alzheimer's Disease: Inside Looking Out." 18 min., 1995.
> Terra Nova Films
> 9848 S. Winchester Ave.
> Chicago, IL 60643
> (312) 881-8491

"Voices of Caregiving: Insights from Along the Way." 31 min., 1995.
> Terra Nova Films
> 9848 S. Winchester Ave.
> Chicago, IL 60643
> (312) 881-8491

"Another Home for Mom." 30 min., 1995.
> Fanlight Productions
> 47 Halifax Street
> Boston, MA 02130
> (800) 937-4113

"Living with Alzheimer's": 3-part series. 1995.
> "Understanding Alzheimer's." 35 min.
> "Choices in Caregiving." 35 min.
> "Challenges of Caregiving." 35 min.
>> Long Island Alzheimer's Foundation
>> 99 South Street
>> Patchogue, NY 11772
>> (800) 399-2244

Internet Sites

Alzheimer's Association, National Headquarters	http://www.alz.org
Alzheimer's Association, St. Louis Chapter	http://www.alzstl.org
Alzheimer's Disease Education and Referral Center (ADEAR)	http://www.alzheimers.org/adear
Alzheimer's Disease Research Center	http://www.biostat.wustl.edu/ADCnet
Washington University at St. Louis, Alzheimer Page	http://www.biostat.wustl.edu/ALZHEIMER
Massachusetts General Hospital Genetics and Aging Unit	http://demo0nmac.mgh.harvard.edu/alzheimers/alzheimer.html
Indiana Alzheimer Disease Center National Cell Repository	http://www.hslib.washington.edu/genline/alzheimer.html